Instant Clinical Pharmacology

Instant Clinical Pharmacology

Evan J. Begg

BSc, MB, ChB (Auckland), MD (Otago), FRACP
Professor in Medicine/Clinical Pharmacology
Christchurch School of Medicine
University of Otago
Christchurch
New Zealand

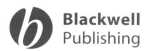
Blackwell
Publishing

First published 2003 by Blackwell Publishing Ltd

ISBN 1-4051-0275-6

Catalogue records for this title are available from the British Library and the Library of Congress

Set in 9/12pt Sabon by Graphicraft Limited, Hong Kong
Printed and bound in Great Britain by MPG Books Ltd, Bodmin, Cornwall

Commissioning Editor: Fiona Goodgame
Production Editor: Julie Elliott
Production Controller: Chris Downs

For further information on Blackwell Publishing, visit our website:
www.blackwellpublishing.com

Contents

Introduction

This book is written mainly for medical students and doctors undergoing postgraduate training. Students of allied health professionals, such as pharmacy, nursing, dentistry and physiotherapy may also find it useful.

The aim is to provide essential information about the core topics in clinical pharmacology. There is general agreement across the world about what constitutes this core curriculum. These topics are covered, the emphasis reflecting my own biases.

The book assumes a knowledge of basic pharmacology and does not embrace specific therapeutics. It aims to bridge the gap between basic pharmacology and the therapeutic use of drugs in humans.

Some readers may be put off by the slightly mathematical nature of the initial section on clinical pharmacokinetics. I apologize for this, but unfortunately this is the basis of clinical pharmacology. The book gets easier after this.

Any feedback would be appreciated, particularly in terms of improving the user-friendliness of the book.

I acknowledge with warm gratitude the input and inspiration of all the members of my department, both past and present. The book is dedicated to my students, whose humour and wide-eyed enthusiasm makes teaching so worthwhile.

How to use the book

Mindful of the fickle nature of the learning process, I have tried to keep things simple and to encapsulate each topic within two facing pages. Hopefully, this will enable the reader to complete a topic in a short learning session before the inevitable build-up of boredom!

Happy learning!

Evan J. Begg

What is Clinical Pharmacology?

Clinical pharmacology is concerned with the rational, safe and effective use of medicines.

Clinical pharmacology
The principles behind the prescribing process

as opposed to

Therapeutics
The process of medical treatment

Clinical pharmacology involves the complex interaction between the **patient** and the **drug**. The patient is a unique individual, with many distinguishing features that need to be taken into account during prescribing. The patient can be described in terms of the **patient profile**. The drug, likewise, is unique, with its own distinguishing features. It may be described in terms of the **drug profile**.

Good prescribing involves tailoring the drug and dosing regimen to the unique patient. Clinical pharmacology provides the basis of this.

Patient profile	Drug profile
Age	Name (generic)
Weight	Class
Sex	Action
Race	Pharmacokinetics
Allergies	Indications
Smoking history	Contraindications/
Alcohol history	precautions
Diseases	Interactions
Pregnant/lactating	Side effects
Current therapy	Dosing regimen
Intelligence	Monitoring
	Overdose

For example, once a diagnosis has been made and drug therapy is considered appropriate, a particular drug must be chosen. The ideal drug is chosen, based on the best evidence. This drug is then examined to see if it is appropriate for *this* patient.
- Is the patient allergic to this drug or class?
- Are there any potential interactions with the patient's other drugs?
- Does the patient have other diseases that might be made worse (or better) by the addition of the new drug?
- Is compliance likely to be a problem?

If the drug passes this first test, then a dosage regimen must be chosen. The starting point is the 'normal' dose regimen that would be appropriate for the 'average' patient. This dosage regimen is then adjusted to tailor it to *this* patient.
- Is the patient old? (may need a lower dose)
- Is there any renal impairment/liver impairment? (may need a lower dose or a longer dose interval)
- Are there any drug interactions that might require dose alteration?

Problems with these 'ideals'

It is easy to preach a 'holier than thou' approach to therapeutics, but harder to achieve this in practice. Individualizing drugs to the patient may be different in different settings. Prescribing in outback Australia is likely to be very different from prescribing in central Sydney. Access to laboratories and medical follow-up will be different. The ideal drug, based on evidence, may be totally impractical for your particular patient.

The 'rational, safe and effective use of medicines' must be tolerant of all this. Prescribers should not be expected to achieve perfection, but to pursue the greatest possible effectiveness, with minimal risks, and to respect the patient's choice. The word 'rational' is relevant here, denoting not only scientific rationality, but also situational rationality.

1 Clinical pharmacokinetics

General Overview of Pharmacokinetics

The aim of drug therapy is to achieve efficacy without toxicity. This involves achieving a plasma concentration (Cp) that is above the *minimal effective concentration* (MEC), but below the *minimal toxic concentration* (MTC).

Clinical pharmacokinetics is about all the factors that determine the Cp and its time-course, i.e. it is about variability. The various factors are dealt with in subsequent chapters.

Constant IV infusion

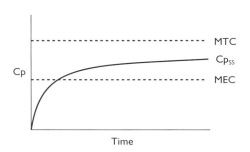

The Cp rises to reach the desired steady state concentration (Cp$_{SS}$). The main determinant of the Cp$_{SS}$ is the dose and the clearance (Cl).

Loading dose (IV injection followed by a constant infusion)

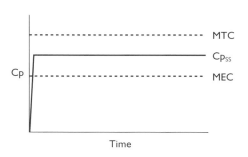

In order to achieve early effect (e.g. treating status epilepticus with phenytoin) it is important to get the Cp up to the effect zone as soon as possible. This is achieved with a loading dose.

The factor determining the loading dose is the volume of distribution (Vd).

Oral dosing

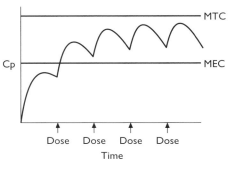

The curve reflects assimilation and elimination, and intermittent administration.

Cp higher than desired

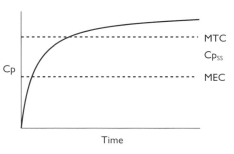

The two factors involved are excessive dosage and/or decreased Cl.

Factors causing decreased Cl are:
- normal variation
- saturable metabolism
- genetic enzyme deficiency
- renal failure
- liver failure
- old age
- very young age (neonate)
- enzyme inhibition.

Cp lower than desired

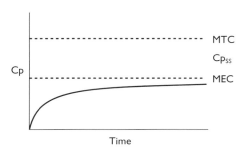

Dose may be too low, or Cl too high. Factors causing increased Cl are:
- normal variation
- poor absorption
- high first-pass metabolism
- genetic hypermetabolism
- enzyme induction
- non-compliance.

Time to steady state

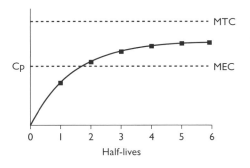

This is determined by the $t_{1/2}$ of the drug. It takes $4 \times t_{1/2}$ to achieve >90% of the steady-state concentration.

Time for drug elimination

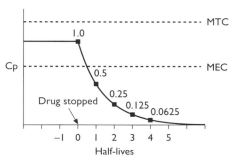

This is determined by the $t_{1/2}$ of the drug. It takes $4 \times t_{1/2}$ for concentrations to reduce to <10% of the starting value.

Components of the line of steady state

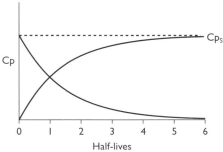

The line of steady state is effectively made up of the sum of the line of accumulation and the line of elimination. i.e. the net effect of input and output.

3

Pharmacokinetics

> **Pharmacokinetics:**
> The study of the **movement** of drugs into,
> within and out of the body
> i.e. **what the body does to the drug**

as opposed to

> **Pharmacodynamics:**
> The study of drug **effect**, and
> mechanisms of action
> i.e. **what the drug does to the body**

It is important to know the pharmacokinetics of a drug so that the drug can be used in a rational and scientific manner, and the dose tailored to the patient.

The most important pharmacokinetic parameters from a dosing point of view are the clearance (Cl), the volume of distribution (Vd) and the half-life of elimination ($t_{1/2}$). The Cl determines the maintenance dose, the Vd the loading dose, and the $t_{1/2}$ the dose interval.

One-compartment model

The most simple model is the one-compartment model. In this, the body is considered as a single container (one compartment) in which the drug is instantaneously and uniformly distributed.

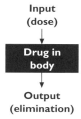

**Input
(dose)**

**Drug in
body**

**Output
(elimination)**

Pharmacokinetics involves the study of the movement of the drug into, within and out of the body. From a dosing point of view it is the concentration of drug at the site of action that is important. This is difficult to measure. Under steady-state conditions the plasma concentration (Cp) is in equilibrium with sites of action. In practice it is usually the Cp that is measured.

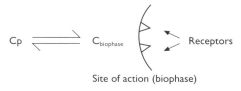

$$Cp \rightleftharpoons C_{biophase} \quad \rightarrow \quad Receptors$$

Site of action (biophase)

The pharmacokinetics of a drug are usually studied using an intravenous injection or infusion, as the dose can then be considered to be 100% assimilated into the body. The values of Cl, Vd and $t_{1/2}$ for a drug are derived from the curve of concentration versus time.

Zero-order elimination

It would be very simple if the Cp declined linearly with time after a simple intravenous injection. This situation, called *zero-order* elimination, occurs only rarely. A familiar example is ethanol, concentrations of which decline at a constant rate of approximately 15 mg/100 mL/h.

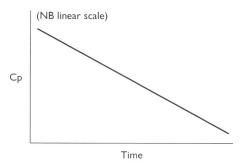

(NB linear scale)

Cp

Time

First-order elimination

The more common situation is *first-order* elimination, in which the decline in plasma concentrations is not constant with time, but varies with the concentration. The higher the concentration, the greater the rate of elimination. The concentration declines 'exponentially' with time.

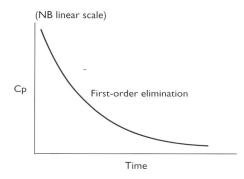

This curve can be described by:
$$Cp_t = Cp_o * e^{-kt}$$

where Cp_t is the concentration at any time t
Cp_o is the concentration at time zero
and   k is the elimination rate constant

This equation is difficult to use (for most of us!) and can be simplified by transforming it to a linear expression. This is done by taking the natural logarithm of each side:

$$\ln Cp_t = \ln Cp_o - kt$$

This now has the form of a linear equation $y = mx + c$, or in this case because the line is declining, $y = c - mx$, where m is the slope and c the intercept on the y-axis.

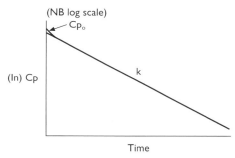

Important pharmacokinetic abbreviations

Abbreviation	Definition	Abbreviation	Definition
$t_{1/2}$	the half-life of elimination	ss	**S**teady **s**tate
Vd	**V**olume of **d**istribution	Cp	**P**lasma **c**oncentration
Cl	**Cl**earance	Cp_t	**P**lasma **c**oncentration at **t**ime = **t**
AUC	**A**rea **u**nder the **c**urve	Cp_o	**P**lasma **c**oncentration at time = **o**
F	**F**ractional oral availability	Cp_{ss}	**P**lasma **c**oncentration at **s**teady **s**tate
fu	**f**raction excreted **u**nchanged	Ab	**A**mount in **b**ody
PB	**P**rotein **B**inding	e	The natural logarithm
T_{max}	**T**ime to **max**imum concentration		(value = 2.7183)
C_{max}	Peak concentration	ln	log to the base e
	(**C**oncentration **max**imum)	k	the rate constant of elimination

|

Drug Clearance

> **Drug clearance (from plasma)** is defined as:
> 'The volume of plasma cleared of drug
> per unit time';
> or
> 'A constant relating the rate of elimination to
> the plasma concentration (Cp)'
> i.e. rate of elimination = Cl * Cp
> Units: vol/time (e.g. L/h)

Clearance (Cl) is the single most important pharmacokinetic parameter. Cl determines the **maintenance dose-rate**, i.e. dose per unit time, required to *maintain* a plasma concentration.

Clearance does not apply to drugs with zero-order kinetics, but only to those with first-order (exponential) kinetics. This applies to the majority of drugs.

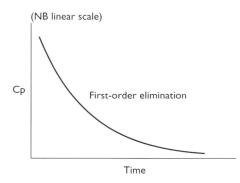

(NB linear scale)

Cp

First-order elimination

Time

The graph shows that the rate of elimination (RE) is different at different concentrations, i.e. it is *driven* by concentration.

rate of elimination ∝ Cp
∴ rate of elimination (mg/h) = constant
(L/h) * Cp (mg/L)

This 'constant' is the **clearance** (Cl) and by deduction has units of volume/time (e.g. L/h), since the units for rate of elimination are mg/h, and for concentration mg/L.

> i.e. rate of elimination = Cl * Cp

Thus, Cl is 'A constant relating the rate of elimination to the plasma concentration'; and
'The volume of plasma cleared of drug per unit time'.

The equation can be rearranged as follows:

$$Cl \ (L/h) = \frac{\text{rate of elimination (mg/h)}}{Cp \ (mg/l)}$$

Achievement of a constant steady-state plasma drug concentration (Cp_{SS})

In order to maintain a target Cp, the drug must be administered at a rate equal to the rate of elimination at that concentration, i.e.

rate of administration = rate of elimination
Since
rate of elimination   = Cl * Cp, then
rate of administration = Cl * Cp_{SS}, or

> Maintenance dose-rate = Cl * Cp_{SS}

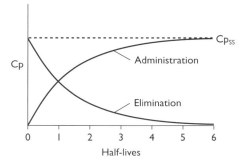

Cp

Cp_{SS}

Administration

Elimination

0   1   2   3   4   5   6
Half-lives

Physiological relevance of drug clearance

The main organs responsible for drug clearance are the liver (metabolism) and the kidneys (removal of unchanged drug). Total body Cl is the sum of all clearance processes, i.e.

Cl (total) = Cl (renal) + Cl (liver) +
                Cl (other)

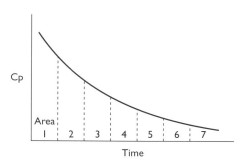

Determination of Cl

Plasma Cl is usually determined from the area under the plasma concentration vs time curve (AUC) after IV administration.

The AUC is determined using the 'trapezoidal rule'.

AUC = Area 1 + Area 2 + Area 3 + . . . Area n, where each area is approximated by a trapezium.

Area under the curve (AUC)

The bigger the AUC, the smaller the Cl.

$$Cl = \frac{Dose}{AUC}$$

After oral administration:

$$Cl = \frac{F * Dose}{AUC}$$

where F = oral availability.

7

Volume of Distribution

> The **volume of distribution** is:
> 'The volume into which a drug appears
> to be distributed with a concentration
> equal to that of plasma,'
> or
> 'A proportionality constant relating
> the plasma concentration (Cp) to the
> amount of drug in the body (Ab).'
> i.e. $Ab = Vd * Cp$
> Units: Volume or vol/kg

The volume of distribution (Vd) is the second most important pharmacokinetic parameter (after Cl). It determines the **loading dose**, i.e. the dose required to achieve a target plasma concentration (Cp) as soon as possible.

In order to achieve a target Cp, the tissues into which the drug distributes (i.e. the volume of distribution) must be 'filled up'.

The Vd is therefore 'the volume into which a drug appears to be distributed with a concentration equal to that of plasma'.

After distribution is complete, the amount of drug in the body (Ab) is proportional to the plasma concentration (Cp).

i.e. $Ab \propto Cp$

or $Ab = constant * Cp$

This constant has units of volume (e.g. L) since the Ab is in mass units (e.g. mg) and Cp is in concentration units (e.g. mg/L).

Hence the Vd is 'A proportionality constant relating the plasma concentration to the amount of drug in the body.'

i.e. $Ab = Vd * cp$

or $Vd = \dfrac{Ab}{Cp}$

The Vd is often called the 'apparent' Vd since the volume has no real anatomical meaning. This can be appreciated when the volume of the body (50–100 L) is compared with Vds of drugs, e.g. heparin (5 L); gentamicin (15 L); digoxin (500 L); and quinacrine (20 000 L).

Highly lipid soluble drugs such as quinacrine have much larger Vds than very polar, water soluble drugs such as heparin.

Determination of Vd

To calculate Vd, the Ab and Cp need to be known. The only time Ab is known accurately is immediately after the drug has been given intravenously (prior to elimination), i.e. the dose. If the Cp at time zero (Cp_0) is known, then the Vd can be calculated. The Cp_0 can be determined from the lnCp vs time curve after intravenous (IV) administration. After initial distribution, there is a 'log-linear' decline in plasma concentration. The Cp_0 can be determined by back-extrapolating the linear portion of the curve to its intercept on the y-axis. Vd can then be calculated.

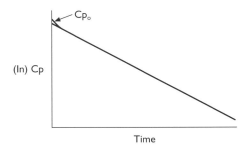

i.e.   At time zero,   Ab   = dose
                         then   dose = $Vd * Cp_0$
                         or   Vd   = $dose/Cp_0$

Calculation of loading dose (LD)

It follows from the above that to achieve a target Cp, the Vd of the drug must be known

$$LD = Vd * target\ Cp$$

e.g. to achieve a target Cp of digoxin (Vd ~ 500 L) of 1.5 µg/L, a loading dose (LD) of 750 µg, or 0.75 mg is needed, i.e.

LD (µg) = 500 (L) * 1.5 (µg/L)
        = 750 µg

With a loading dose, steady-state concentrations can be achieved quickly.

Curve A — loading dose followed by maintenance dosing.
Curve B — maintenance dosing every half-life.

In summary, the most important thing about Vd is that it enables the calculation of a loading dose to achieve any desired Cp.

$$LD = Vd * Cp$$

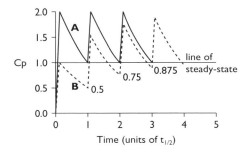

The Half-Life

The **half-life of elimination** ($t_{1/2}$) is:
'The time for the concentration of
the drug in plasma (or the amount of
drug in the body) to halve.'
Units: Time (usually h)

The $t_{1/2}$ provides an index of:
1 the time-course of drug elimination;
2 the time-course of drug accumulation; and
3 choice of dose interval.

Derivation of $t_{1/2}$

The half-life of elimination ($t_{1/2}$) can be
derived by plotting actual concentrations on
semilog graph paper, or logged concentrations on linear graph paper. It is the time
taken for any concentration to halve, e.g.
from 3 to 1.5 mg/L.

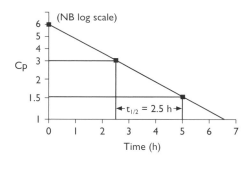

Time-course of drug elimination

If a drug is discontinued after an infusion,
the Cp will decline exponentially to <10% of
its starting value after four half-lives.

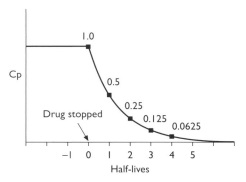

Time-course of drug accumulation

If a drug is started as a constant infusion, the
Cp will accumulate to approach steady-state
(>90% of steady state concentration) after
four half-lives.

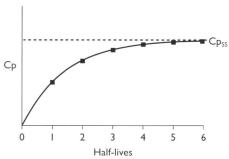

Components of the line of steady state

The line of steady state is effectively the combination of accumulation and elimination. i.e. it is the sum of the effect of dose and elimination at any time point.

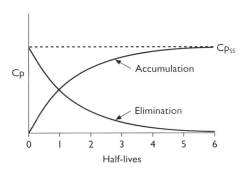

Choice of dose interval

The dose interval is usually chosen based on:
1 the $t_{1/2}$
2 the therapeutic index of the drug
3 compliance — it is best, if possible, to have dosing once or twice a day.
If drug Cl decreases (say in renal dysfunction), it may be possible for a drug that is normally given three or four times a day to be given twice or once daily, with greater chance of compliance. This is good therapeutics.

Relationship between $t_{1/2}$, Vd and Cl

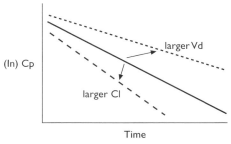

It is logical that the larger the Vd, the longer the $t_{1/2}$, i.e. it takes longer to remove drug from deep within the tissues. Similarly, it is logical that the larger the Cl, the shorter the $t_{1/2}$. In other words:

$$t_{1/2} \propto \frac{Vd}{Cl}$$

This relationship can be turned into an equation by multiplying the right side by 0.693. This strange number is the natural logarithm of 2 (i.e. ln 2) and gets into the equation because the $t_{1/2}$ involves a halving, i.e. the inverse of 2.

$$t_{1/2} = \frac{0.693Vd}{Cl}$$

This is one of the most important equations in clinical pharmacokinetics.
• It indicates that the $t_{1/2}$ is *dependent* on Vd and Cl.
• Vd and Cl are the *independent* variables.

Oral Availability

Oral availability is:
The fraction of drug that reaches the systemic circulation after oral ingestion

Oral availability defines how much drug gets 'on board' after oral ingestion. 'Absorption' and 'first-pass' metabolism are the main determinants of oral availability.

Oral availability is usually defined by comparison with the total availability of drug in the systemic circulation after IV dosing, i.e. the fraction (F) of drug that gets into the body after oral (po) versus IV administration:

i.e. $$F = \frac{AUC_{po}}{AUC_{IV}}$$

The total amount of drug in the systemic circulation is defined by the area under the concentration–time curve (AUC). The AUC may be different after oral compared with IV administration. The oral availability may have a value of one, or less than one.

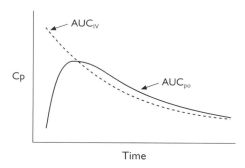

Time

Determinants of oral availability

1 Absorption.
2 First-pass metabolism.

Absorption

This refers to the ability of the drug to cross a biological barrier into the blood. In the case of oral absorption, it refers to crossing the gut wall into the portal circulation. Absorption is usually a passive process governed by the principles of diffusion (i.e. flows down a concentration gradient). Sometimes, active transport is involved (e.g. L-dopa). Factors favouring absorption include high lipid solubility and low ionization. pH may also influence absorption, but probably affects the rate more than the extent.

First-pass metabolism

This refers to metabolism of the drug prior to reaching the systemic circulation, i.e. *presystemic elimination*. Some drugs, such as highly lipid-soluble drugs, are so highly metabolized that on 'first-pass' through the liver there is substantial 'presystemic' elimination. Presystemic elimination can occur in the gut wall (e.g. oestrogens), in the portal circulation (e.g. aspirin → salicylic acid) or in the liver (the majority).

Effect of food on oral availability

Interestingly, food affects absorption and first-pass metabolism in opposite ways. Food usually *decreases* the oral availability of sparingly lipid-soluble drugs that are subject to absorptive problems, e.g. food decreases the oral availability of atenolol by 50%.

However, food usually increases the oral availability of drugs that are subject to high first-pass metabolism. This is because food increases portal venous blood flow, thereby increasing the presentation of absorbed drug to the liver, partially saturating metabolizing pathways and opening up shunts that by-pass metabolizing pathways. The net result is *greater* oral availability, e.g. food increases the oral availability of metoprolol by 50%.

Some foods, e.g. grapefruit juice, compete with drugs for presystemic elimination, thereby causing increased oral availability of the drug (e.g. calcium antagonists, some statins).

Confusing terminology

There is sometimes confusion between the terms 'oral *availability*', 'bioavailability' and 'absorption'. Oral availability is the preferred term because it is unambiguous.

'Bioavailability' has a strict historical definition — 'the **rate** and **extent** of *absorption*'. One problem with 'bioavailability' is its reference to absorption. As noted above, absorption is only one part of the process of drug attaining the systemic circulation. The other problem with 'bioavailability' is that it is a single term that defines two processes — the *rate* of absorption, and the *extent*. It is more instructive to think of each of these components independently, i.e. oral availability defines the *extent*, and another term, T_{max}, defines the *rate*.

Time to peak concentration (T_{max})

> T_{max} defines the time to **max**imum (or peak) concentration

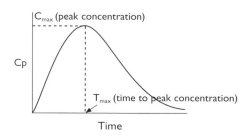

T_{max} is less important than the total oral availability. A short T_{max} may be useful where an immediate effect is desired, e.g. analgesia for a headache. A short T_{max} may also be a problem e.g. adverse effects related to the peak concentration.

Slow-release preparations

A delayed T_{max} and a longer drug action may be achieved using tablets or capsules designed to release their contents slowly. This flattens the concentration–time profile, giving a more even drug response.

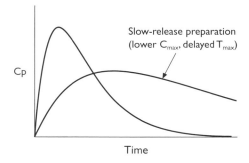

Protein Binding

The major message about protein binding (PB) is that it is usually not important.

> Protein binding is only important in the interpretation of measured plasma concentrations

There is enormous confusion about the importance of protein binding and the drug effects attributed to it. While drugs may displace each other from protein-binding sites, this is almost always unimportant. Most alleged protein binding interactions of clinical importance have an additional mechanism operating, such as altered drug clearance, that is the reason underlying the observed clinical effects.

Acidic drugs bind largely to albumin. Basic drugs bind mainly to α_1-acid glycoprotein (i.e. orosomucoid), an acute phase reactant, and to albumin and β-lipoproteins.

The significance of protein binding lies in the interpretation of plasma concentrations of drugs. If plasma concentrations are not measured, protein binding can largely be ignored.

NB: When plasma concentrations of drugs are measured, it is *total drug*, i.e. bound + unbound, that is measured. It is possible, but not routine (except perhaps for phenytoin), to measure free or unbound drug.

Measured drug

Bound drug $\rightleftharpoons$ Free drug

Altered albumin or α_1-acid glycoprotein concentrations will alter the measured (total) concentrations of drugs bound highly to these proteins.

However, it is free drug that acts on receptors to produce effect. Therefore, it is the concentration of free drug, not total drug, that is actually important in terms of desired effects and side effects.

Free drug concentration is dependent on free drug clearance (see Clearance, page 6), and does not vary in relation to changes in plasma proteins. Therefore, except for rare exceptions, no alteration in dosage is required in states of altered protein binding.

The fallacy of protein-binding drug interactions

Many so-called protein-binding drug interactions have been reported. While drugs can compete for protein binding sites, especially on albumin, this does not affect the free concentration.

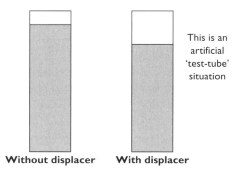

This is an artificial 'test-tube' situation

Without displacer   **With displacer**

If a drug in the body was not subject to drug elimination, then introduction of a protein-binding displacer would increase the concentration of the free drug.

In reality drug elimination does occur. Since the steady-state free drug concentration is only dependent on maintenance dose and free drug clearance (remember, Maintenance dose = Cl * Cp), then free drug concentration returns to its predisplacement level. However, the total drug concentration is now lower than it was.

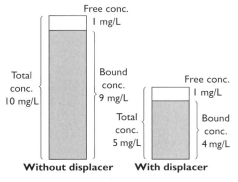

Without displacer   With displacer

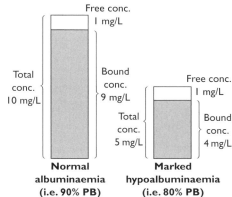

Normal
albuminaemia
(i.e. 90% PB)

Marked
hypoalbuminaemia
(i.e. 80% PB)

Interpretation of measured plasma concentrations during therapeutic drug monitoring

Protein binding 'problems' arise from the fact that the measured drug concentration is total drug (bound + unbound). In hypoalbuminaemia (e.g. in renal disease) an acidic drug such as phenytoin will have a lower total drug concentration because of lower protein binding. Free drug concentration will, however, be the same as in the non-hypoalbuminaemic state (assuming free drug Cl is constant). The same principles apply with displacing drugs in normoalbuminaemia. e.g. *phenytoin* (therapeutic range 10–20 mg/L total concentration, 1–2 mg/L free concentration).

In hypoalbuminaemia free concentration (and effect) is identical but total measured concentration is half. If the dose was increased to give a total concentration of 10 mg/L, the free concentration would be 2 mg/L and may be toxic. Note that the situation for hypoalbuminaemia is identical to that involving drug displacement interactions (see above).

Drugs with saturable protein binding

Some drugs at clinical concentrations saturate the available protein-binding sites. In this situation total drug concentration (bound + unbound) does not increase linearly with dose. Interpretation of measured concentrations is difficult. If free concentrations were measured, these would be seen to rise linearly with dose.

Drugs with saturable protein binding include ceftriaxone, hydrocortisone, prednisone, thioridazine and sodium valproate. Of these, the only one that has clinical importance is sodium valproate, because this is sometimes measured during therapeutic drug monitoring. Saturable protein binding makes interpretation of valproate concentrations difficult. For the other drugs protein binding does not need to be taken into account during dosing, because drug concentrations are not usually measured, and free concentrations behave predictably.

pH and Pharmacokinetics

In some situations drug disposition varies in relation to pH differences across biological barriers. The disposition of some weak acids and bases is susceptible to small pH differences because of variation in the state of ionization and hence the ability to cross membranes.

Background theory

> Acids are ionized in basic media
> Bases are ionized in acidic media

i.e. $H^+ + X^- \rightleftharpoons HX$

   (ionized)   (unionized)

If more H^+ ions are added (i.e. adding acidity), the equilibrium moves to the right. If base (e.g. OH^-) is added, H^+ ions are consumed, and the equilibrium moves to the left. Unionized drug crosses lipid biological barriers (e.g. membranes) better than ionized drug.

Henderson–Hasselbalch equation

For acids:

$$pH = pK_a + \log_{10} \times \left(\frac{[\text{ionized}]}{[\text{unionized}]} \right)$$

For bases:

$$pH = pK_a + \log_{10} \times \left(\frac{[\text{unionized}]}{[\text{ionized}]} \right)$$

NB The pK_a is the pH at which a drug is 50% ionized and 50% unionized. Weak acids, with pK_a values between 3 and 7.5, may show variation in the ionized/unionized ratio at pHs encountered in physiology. Similarly, weak bases with pK_a values between 5 and 11 may show variation in the unionized/ionized ratio.

When is this important?

- Drug absorption from the stomach
- Drug elimination via the kidneys
- Drug distribution into milk
- Drug distribution across the placenta.

Drug absorption from the stomach

Gastric pH is usually between 1 and 4. Acids are therefore largely unionized and may be absorbed in the stomach (e.g. aspirin). However, because of the far greater absorptive surface area in the small intestine, the bulk of absorption occurs there, even for acids.

Drug elimination in the kidney

The pH in the urine varies from 4.5 to 7.5. Weak acids may vary from unionized at pH 4.5 to largely ionized at pH 7.5. Reabsorption from the renal tubular lumen into the blood will occur if the drug is in the unionized state. Therefore, reabsorption will occur in acid urine, while elimination will occur in alkaline urine. Conversely, weak bases will be reabsorbed in alkaline urine and eliminated in acid urine. This principle is sometimes used in enhancing the elimination of drugs after overdoses (e.g. aspirin elimination can be enhanced by administration of bicarbonate).

Drugs with pH-dependent elimination

Acids (elimination enhanced by alkaline diuresis)
• phenobarbitone
• salicylates.

Bases (elimination enhanced by acid diuresis)
• amphetamines
• methadone
• mexiletine
• phencyclidine
• phenylpropanolamines (e.g. ephedrine, pseudoephedrine)
• quinidine.

Drug distribution into milk, across the placenta, and into '3rd spaces'

Milk, the fetus, and most '3rd spaces' have pH values that are acidic (~7.0) in relation to plasma (~7.4). Therefore bases tend to concentrate in these 'compartments' because they are relatively ionized on the acidic side, and effectively 'trapped'. This is called 'ion trapping'. It applies to any situation where a pH gradient exists across a biological barrier, and where the principles of diffusion apply, e.g. abscesses, synovial fluid.

2 Factors affecting dosing

Drug Metabolism

Variation in drug metabolism is a major cause of variation in drug clearance

Some drugs are excreted unchanged through the kidneys because they are polar and are not reabsorbed in the renal tubules. Other drugs, especially those that are lipid-soluble, are reabsorbed in the renal tubules and would circulate forever if they were not biotransformed to more readily excretable forms.

Metabolic biotransformation converts drugs to more polar and excretable forms. The resulting metabolite may be inactive, less active or occasionally more active (e.g. metabolite of a prodrug) than the parent molecule.

Where does biotransformation occur?

Metabolism occurs mainly in the liver, but also in the kidney, lung, GI mucosa, plasma, the CNS and probably most tissues. Some drugs undergo sequential biotransformation.

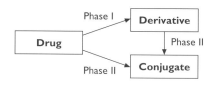

Phase I reactions include oxidation, reduction and hydrolysis. The most common are *oxidation* reactions (adding oxygen, or removing hydrogen). Oxidation reactions include dealkylation, hydroxylation, deamination and desulphuration. Most occur via the cytochrome p450 enzymes.

Phase II reactions involve conjugations, such as glucuronidation, acetylation, sulphation and methylation. Glucuronidation is quantitatively the most important.

Cytochrome R450 metabolism (CYP)

CYP reactions are catalysed by the cytochrome p450 mixed function oxidases, mostly in the liver. These are iron-containing enzymes, named p for pigment, and 450 for the wavelength, in nM, at which spectrophotometric absorption occurs. At least 13 CYP gene families exist in humans, with various subfamilies. Each CYP family is encoded by a separate gene. The nomenclature is:

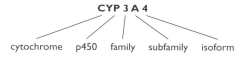

Drug clearance by the liver

The fraction of drug removed from blood in one passage across the liver is the extraction ratio (ER).

$$ER = \frac{C_{in} - C_{out}}{C_{in}}$$

where C = drug concentration

Hepatic drug clearance depends on the extraction ratio, but also on the hepatic blood flow (HBF) since the greater the blood flow the greater the presentation of drug to the liver. Thus,

Hepatic Cl = HBF * ER

High Cl, flow-dependent elimination: If the extraction ratio approaches 1 (complete extraction), then hepatic Cl approaches hepatic blood flow. In this case the elimination is said to be 'blood flow dependent', or 'high clearance'.

Low Cl, flow-independent elimination: If the extraction ratio is small, there is no blood flow dependence, since presentation of more drug to the liver will not result in greater elimination.

First-pass metabolism: Drugs entering the portal system after absorption have to pass through the liver prior to reaching the systemic circulation. If the extraction ratio approaches 1, little drug will reach the systemic circulation. In this case, 'first-pass' elimination approaches 100%, and oral availability (F) approaches zero. For example, lignocaine has an extraction ratio of 0.7, and therefore an F of 0.3.

There are three situations in which the extent of first-pass metabolism decreases, resulting in increased oral availability:

1 High oral doses — Drugs such as propranolol saturate the metabolizing enzymes, resulting in less first-pass metabolism, and greater oral availability.

2 High blood flow — Increased liver blood flow, such as after food, delivers more drug to the metabolizing enzymes, sometimes saturating them. This results in less first-pass metabolism for high clearance drugs such as propranolol.

3 Chronic liver disease — There is lower intrinsic clearance, as well as increased shunting.

Some examples of high and low clearance drugs.

High clearance	Low clearance
Antidepressants	NSAIDs
Antipsychotics	Anticonvulsants
Calcium antagonists	Most benzodiazepines
Narcotics	
Nitrates	
Most antiparkinson's	
Most statins	
Many β-blockers	

Clinical significance of high-clearance drugs

- Subject to first-pass metabolism
- Subject to flow-dependent elimination
- May require dose-reduction in situations of decreased blood flow, e.g. congestive heart failure (CHF)
- May be subject to pre-systemic drug interactions, e.g. with grapefruit juice.

Saturable Metabolism

Saturable metabolism causes drug concentrations to rise disproportionately (non-linearly) compared with dose

It is theoretically possible for all drugs to saturate their metabolizing pathways. For most drugs the concentration at which saturation begins to be evident is usually above the concentration range used in therapeutics. For a few drugs, however, saturation occurs at therapeutic concentrations.

Consider the Michaelis–Menten curve:

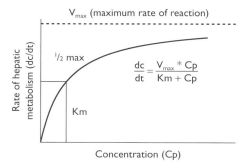

The curve asymptotes to a maximum *rate* of reaction (V_{max}). The Km (Michaelis constant) is the *concentration* at which half the maximum rate of reaction occurs.

$$\frac{dc}{dt} = \frac{V_{max} * Cp}{Km + Cp}$$

V_{max} relates to the total amount of enzymes available for metabolism. Km is inversely proportional to the affinity of the drug for the enzyme, i.e. the higher the affinity the lower the Km.

Enzyme inducers, which increase the amount of available enzymes, will therefore increase V_{max} but will not alter Km.

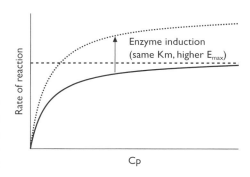

Enzyme inhibitors which act by competing with other drugs for metabolism by the same enzyme, will not change the V_{max}, but will increase the Km. Enzyme inhibitors that act by direct inhibition of the enzyme will decrease the V_{max} and may or may not alter the Km.

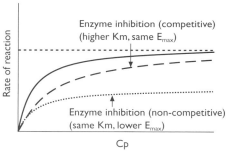

NB Below the Km, the rate of elimination is almost directly proportional to the plasma concentration (i.e. RE $\propto$ Cp. This is equivalent to Cp to the first power, or 'first order'). This is therefore a 'first-order' reaction, and graphically is a straight line if log Cp is plotted against T.

Above the Km, the rate of elimination becomes independent of concentration. This is called 'zero-order' elimination because it is not dependent on Cp (equivalent to Cp^o where any number to the power of zero equals 1).

In practice, most drugs have Km values well above their therapeutic concentrations, and therefore have first-order kinetics.

A select group of well-known drugs saturate at or around their therapeutic concentrations. For these, concentrations may increase more than proportionally for a given increase in dose, e.g. *phenytoin*.

- Aspirin saturates after only one or two 300 mg tablets.
- Alcohol has a Km of approximately 0.01 g/100 mL, and therefore metabolism is essentially zero order at almost all concentrations (usual driving limits 0.05–0.08 g/ 100 mL).

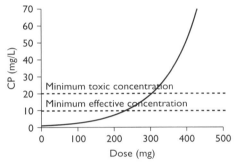

• Phenytoin has a Km of around 7 mg/L and therefore saturates at or around the lower end of the therapeutic range (10–20 mg/L).

Some drugs with non-linear elimination (i.e. dose-dependent, saturable).

Drug	Pathway
alcohol	alcohol dehydrogenase
aspirin	various conjugations
clonidine	active renal tubular excretion
fluoxetine	CYP2D6
methotrexate	active renal tubular excretion
paroxetine	CYP2D6
phenytoin	CYP2C9/2C19
propafenone	CYP2D6
verapamil	CYP3A4

For drugs with saturable elimination dose increases should be made in small increments

Pharmacogenetics

> Some pathways of drug metabolism are affected by genetic polymorphism, with marked dosing implications

Fast/slow acetylation

Acetylation is a phase II conjugation re-action catalysed by *N*-acetyl transferase. Among Caucasians, approximately 50% are fast and 50% are slow acetylators. Acetylation status is determined by parent/metabolite ratios in the plasma or urine. Drugs affected by acetylator status include:
- procainamide and hydralazine (increased risk of SLE in slow acetylators)
- sulphonamides (increased risk of haemolysis in slow acetylators)
- isoniazid (increased risk of peripheral neuropathy in slow acetylators; increased risk of hepatitis in fast acetylators).

Glucuronidation

Glucuronidation, the other major phase II reaction, is also subject to genetic polymorphism. Patients with Gilbert's disease have deficient glucuronyl transferase, reflected by higher bilirubin concentrations.

Aldehyde dehydrogenase

Around 50% of persons of Mongoloid descent have aldehyde dehydrogenase deficiency. They are unable to metabolize acetaldehyde produced from ethanol and may develop a 'disulfiram reaction' — build-up of acetaldehyde causing flushing and vomiting.

Pseudocholinesterase deficiency

One in 3000 individuals cannot metabolize succinylcholine and require artificial respiration for some hours after succinylcholine usage (e.g. during anaesthesia).

Thiopurine methyl transferase (TPMT)

Azathioprine and its metabolite 6-mercap-topurine (6-MP) are metabolized to a variety of active and inactive products. In patients with TPMT deficiency, 6-MP is shunted down alternative pathways, increasing both efficacy and adverse effects, especially bone marrow depression. One in 300 Caucasians are essentially without TPMT activity, while 10% have intermediate activity.

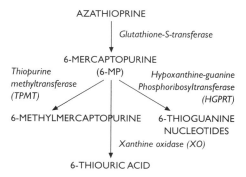

Dihydropyrimidine dehydrogenase (DPD)

5-fluorouracil is metabolized by DPD. Absolute and partial DPD deficiency occurs in around 0.1–3% of the Caucasian population, and in these patients excessive toxicity may be observed.

Cytochrome P450 metabolism (CYP)

The most important isoforms for drug metabolism are CYP3A4, CYP2D6, CYP2C19, CYP2C9, CYP1A2 and CYP2E1. Of these, only CYP2D6, CYP2C9 and CYP2C19 have clearcut and clinically important genetic polymorphisms. More will undoubtably be found, however.

Cytochrome P450 (CYP) polymorphism

The first evidence of CYP polymorphism was the discovery of 'slow hydroxylation' of sparteine and debrisoquine. Both are mediated by CYP2D6. Around 40% of CYP metabolism is carried out by polymorphic enzymes. Interestingly, the major CYP group, CYP3A4, does not appear to be subject to genetic polymorphism.

Determination of CYP status

CYP status may be determined by examining the phenotype (metabolic ratio) or the genotype. The metabolic ratio is the ratio of the parent drug to the metabolite.

CYP2D6

Homozygotes and heterozygotes exist, with appropriate fast and intermediate metabolic ratios. Total absence of the gene results in 'slow metabolism'. There may also be gene duplication or multiple copies resulting in ultrarapid metabolism and very low drug concentrations.

Five to ten per cent of Caucasians and 1–3% of Mongoloid, Polynesian and Negroid people are poor metabolizers. Clinically relevant examples of CYP2D6 poor metabolism include:

- *Perhexiline* — neuropathy/liver toxicity
- *Phenformin* — lactic acidosis
- *Timolol eye drops* — systemic β-blockade
- *Flecainide* — ? arrhythmic deaths.

Codeine requires CYP2D6 to be metabolized to its active metabolite morphine. Since poor CYP2D6 metabolizers have no active CYP2D6 enzyme, codeine does not relieve pain in these patients.

CYP2C9

Around 1–3% of patients on warfarin require only around 1 mg per day for clinical anticoagulation (cf a mean of 7 mg/day in normals), due to poor metabolism.

CYP2C19

Eighteen to 23% of Mongoloid and 3–5% of Caucasian and Negroid people are slow metabolizers. The area under the curve (AUC) of omeprazole (a proton pump inhibitor [PPI]) is increased around 12-fold in patients with slow metabolism.

Characteristics of major CYP drug metabolizing enzymes.

	3A4	2D6	2C9	2C19	1A2	2E1
Chromosome	7	22	10	10	15	10
Probe(s)	Nifedipine	Sparteine Debrisoquine Dextromethorphan	Tolbutamide (Phenytoin)	Mephenytoin	Phenytoin Caffeine	Ethanol
Subject to enzyme induction	++	–	±	±	+	+++
Subject to enzyme inhibition	++	++	+	+	+	±
Subject to genetic polymorphism	No but wide variability	Yes	Yes	Yes	?	?
% of total CYP drugs metabolized by this CYP	50%	25%	5–10%	2–3%	5–10%	5%
Major substrates	Diverse Steroids Ca^{2+} antagonists Macrolides Statins Protease inhibitors	Lipophilic bases Lipophilic β-blockers Antidepressants Neuroleptics Antiarrhythmics Codeine Tramadol	Mainly acids NSAIDs S-warfarin Phenytoin Losartin	Diverse PPIs R-warfarin Phenytoin Moclobemide	Diverse Xanthines Paracetamol	Mainly hydrocarbons Hydrocarbons Anaesthetics

Dosing in Liver Disease and Other Disease States

Liver disease

> The best indices of impaired liver metabolic capacity are a low albumin concentration and raised prothrombin ratio

There is no easily available measure of liver functional impairment (unlike CrCl for renal impairment — see page 28). However, a reduction in drug metabolism in liver disease may occur for three reasons:

1 decreased enzyme metabolizing capacity
2 decreased liver blood flow
3 intra/extra hepatic shunting.

Dosage adjustment may be necessary for extensively metabolized drugs, particularly those with a low therapeutic index.

Drugs with very high metabolic clearance are likely to be affected by decreased blood flow as well as decreased enzyme capacity, and therefore are more susceptible to alterations in liver function.

Some examples of high and low clearance drugs.

High clearance	Low clearance
Antidepressants	NSAIDs
Antipsychotics	Anticonvulsants
Calcium antagonists	Most benzodiazepines
Narcotics	
Nitrates	
Most antiparkinson's	
Most statins	
Many β-blockers	

Assessment of liver impairment

The albumin concentration and the prothrombin indices (such as INR) reflect the ability of the liver to synthesize proteins and therefore are indicative of the liver's ability to synthesize drug metabolizing enzymes. However, these measures are insensitive to rapid changes in liver function and only indicate severe, chronic dysfunction. An albumin concentration of <30 g/L (normal 36–55 g/L) or a raised prothrombin ratio (or INR) indicates severe liver dysfunction.

Chronic liver disease is associated more predictably with impaired metabolism than acute liver disease. Acute liver failure may however be associated with severely impaired drug metabolic capacity.

Diseases of the liver that decrease drug metabolism include: cirrhosis (any cause), alcoholic liver disease, viral hepatitis (may increase or decrease metabolism), porphyria, and hepatoma. Paradoxically, alcoholic liver disease may, if not severe, result in increased metabolism of some drugs through enzyme induction.

NB: Cirrhosis, porphyria and hepatoma do not appear to alter glucuronidation reactions, and therefore drugs solely undergoing glucuronidation are less likely to be affected, e.g. *morphine, lorazepam*.

Cholestatic jaundice

In cholestatic jaundice, drugs or their active metabolites may have impaired elimination if they are extensively cleared unchanged via the bile. In addition, if a drug is cleared as a glucuronide and is subject to enterohepatic cycling (after deconjugation in the gut), this process will be impaired.

Pharmacodynamics

In severe liver disease, hepatic encephalopathy can be precipitated by inappropriate dosing of drugs that cause CNS depression, e.g. sedatives.

Dosing in liver disease

A useful rule, which is somewhat arbitrary, is to:

1 reduce the dose by 50% for high clearance drugs (affected by both blood flow and enzyme capacity).

2 reduce the dose by 25% for low Cl drugs (affected by enzyme capacity only).

Extra caution is advised with drugs with a low therapeutic index. The usual tenet of 'start low, go slow' applies in liver disease. Sometimes it may be more predictable to use glucuronidated rather than oxidized drugs, e.g. lorazepam rather than diazepam, or change to a renally eliminated drug e.g. from metoprolol to atenolol.

> **Dosing in liver disease**
> (if [albumin] <30 g/L or INR elevated)
> • High Cl drugs — ↓ 50%
> • Low Cl drugs — ↓ 25%
> • Change to renally eliminated drug

Cardiovascular disease

The main problem affecting pharmacokinetics is decreased cardiac output (CO), which decreases blood flow to both the liver and the kidney. Effects of decreased cardiac output include:

• Decreased hepatic blood flow causing decreased Cl of high Cl, flow-dependent drugs, e.g. *lignocaine*

• Decreased renal blood flow causing decreased Cl of drugs with high fu, e.g. *digoxin*

• Decreased tissue perfusion causing decreased Vd of lipophilic drugs, e.g. *lignocaine*

• Decreased mesenteric blood flow causing altered rates of absorption, e.g. *frusemide*.

Dosing in cardiovascular disease

The main caution is with high clearance, flow-dependent drugs (see Table). Apply the 'start slow, go slow' strategy. For other drugs, dose in relation to CrCl and albumin/INR status.

Dosing in gastroenterological disease

The small intestine is the most important site of drug absorption. This applies even to acidic drugs, since the huge surface area of the small intestine overshadows other physico-chemical factors (e.g. pK_a, ionization, etc.) which might appear to favour absorption from the stomach. Altered rates of stomach emptying will affect the **RATE** of availability of oral drugs, e.g. migraine → decreased rate of absorption of analgesics.

However, for most drugs the **EXTENT** of availability is more important, and this is rarely altered significantly in GI disease. Diseases most studied have been Crohn's disease, coeliac disease, and gastroenteritis. No simple rules can be made except perhaps that in any circumstance of shortened bowel transit time the potential exists for decreased extent of availability of sparingly soluble or poorly absorbed drugs (e.g. some antibiotics).

Renal Drug Elimination

For drugs that are not metabolized
and are cleared renally unchanged
Drug Cl ∝ CrCl

Some drugs, e.g. *digoxin*, are cleared almost entirely unchanged through the kidneys. Others, e.g. *phenytoin*, are cleared entirely by metabolism. Some prodrugs, e.g. *enalapril*, are converted to active metabolites that are cleared unchanged through the kidneys. Other drugs may be cleared by a combination of the above processes.

Renal clearance of drugs

Glomerular filtration

Drugs pass through the glomerulus where their non-protein-bound component (i.e. free drug) equilibrates across the glomerular membrane. Maximum drug clearance via glomerular filtration alone is therefore equal to the glomerular filtration rate (GFR), i.e. around 1.5 mL/s. Protein binding 'restricts' clearance in proportion to the percentage protein bound, i.e. if protein drug binding is 50%, then drug clearance via glomerular filtration is 50% of the GFR.

Active secretion

Drug not cleared by glomerular filtration continues in the blood to the capillaries adjacent to the proximal renal tubules. Some acids (e.g. penicillins, NSAIDs, probenecid, methotrexate) are actively transported from the blood to the tubular lumen, and subject to energy dependence, saturability, competition, and relative substrate specificity. The process is **not** restricted by protein binding because it is so rapid that drug is easily removed from the protein-binding site. There is also a pathway for basic drugs, e.g. digoxin, dependent on a carrier protein called P-glycoprotein. This is the site of the digoxin–quinidine interaction. An increasing number of drugs are observed to compete at the P-glycoprotein pathway. Active transport enables renal clearance to be larger than the GFR, and theoretically as large as renal blood flow (up to 1500 mL/min).

Reabsorption

Passive reabsorption can occur in the renal tubules. This follows standard principles of diffusion — i.e. depends on concentration gradient, lipid solubility, and sometimes urinary pH (see pH and Pharmacokinetics, page 16). Active reabsorption can occur, e.g. probenecid inhibits the reabsorption of uric acid.

Drug clearance and renal function

For drugs excreted entirely through the kidneys unchanged drug clearance varies in proportion to creatinine clearance (CrCl).

Drug Cl ∝ CrCl

Fraction excreted unchanged (fu)

The fu is the index describing the fraction excreted unchanged through the kidneys. An fu = 1 describes a drug totally cleared renally unchanged. An fu = 0 describes a drug without renal elimination. An fu somewhere in between (e.g. 0.5) describes mixed elimination.

Drug elimination entirely unchanged by the kidney (fu = 1) (e.g. gentamicin)

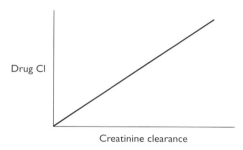

For these drugs, doses should be reduced in direct proportion to the degree of impairment in CrCl. For example, if CrCl is half normal, dose should be half normal.

Drugs eliminated entirely by metabolism (fu = 0) (e.g. phenytoin)

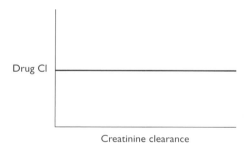

No dose reduction is necessary in renal impairment.

Drug eliminated by both metabolism and by renal elimination (e.g. fu = 0.5) (e.g. captopril)

2

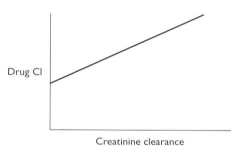

For a drug with fu = 0.5, 50% of the drug is excreted unchanged through the kidneys. If CrCl is half normal, that fraction of the dose should be halved. The metabolized fraction is unaffected, so the total dose should be 75% of normal.

Dosing in Renal Impairment

2

Drugs excreted unchanged through the kidney may need dose alteration in renal impairment

Whenever any active drug moiety is excreted renally unchanged, dose adjustment in relation to renal function may be necessary, especially if the drug has a low therapeutic index.

Dose adjustment in renal impairment

1 Check fu of drug or active metabolite excreted unchanged renally (see Table).

2 Calculate CrCl using an equation such as the Cockcroft & Gault equation* which takes into account the patient's age, weight and sex [use of serum Cr alone is not accurate].

$$CrCl(mL/s) = \frac{(140-age) \times wt[kg]}{50\,000 \times [Cr](mmol/L)}$$

NB: (a) Multiply by 0.85 for females (because of decreased muscle mass)

(b) If patient is obese, use ideal body weight, or an approximation of this

(c) Replace 50 000 by 815 for CrCl in mL/min

* Cockcroft DW, Gault MH. Prediction of creatinine clearance from serum creatinine. *Nephron* 1976, **16**: 31–41.

(d) The equation is not valid for children <12 yrs

(e) Normal CrCl is >1.5 mL/s

(f) If [Cr] is <0.06 mmol/L, use 0.06 in the equation.

3 For drugs **excreted 100% unchanged by the kidneys:**

$$\frac{DR(patient)}{DR(normal)} = \frac{calculated\ CrCl}{1.5}$$

In this case the dose-rate (DR) is decreased in direct proportion to the impairment in renal function (e.g. gentamicin).

4 For drugs **excreted <100% unchanged by the kidneys:**

Obviously dose-adjustment need only be made for that fraction of drug excreted unchanged by the kidney (fu). A general equation that takes into account the fu, the fraction metabolized (1-fu) and the fractional renal function is as follows:

$$\frac{DR(patient)}{DR(normal)} = (1 - fu) + fu \times \left(\frac{calculated\ CrCl}{1.5} \right)$$

5 Should dose be decreased or dose-interval prolonged? The final decision is whether dose adjustment should be by reducing the dose itself or by prolonging the dose-interval. A useful rule is to aim for dosing once or twice a day to allow maximum compliance.

Drugs which may require dose-adjustment in renal impairment.

Low therapeutic index (and fu > 0.5) (Dose-adjustment essential)		**High therapeutic index** (and fu > 0.7) (Dose-adjustment may decrease side effects)	
Drug	**fu**	**Drug**	**fu**
Aminoglycosides		*β-Blockers*	
gentamicin	0.9	atenolol	0.9
tobramycin	0.9	nadolol	0.75
netilmicin	0.9	sotalol	0.9
		bisoprolol	0.6
Cytotoxics			
cisplatin	0.9	*Penicillins*	
carbiplatin	0.9	benzylpenicillin	0.9
methotrexate	0.9–0.5**	amoxycillin	0.9
flucytosine	0.95	(clavulanate)	0.5
		flucloxacillin	0.7
ACE inhibitors		dicloxacillin	0.7
lisinopril	0.9	piperacillin	0.8
enalapril* (enalaprilat)	0.9		
quinapril* (quinaprilat)	0.9	*Cephalosporins*	
cilazapril* (cilazaprilat)	0.9	cephalothin	0.75
ramipril* (ramiprilat)	0.9	cefuroxime	0.9
captopril	0.5	cefaclor	0.7
		cefoxitin	0.8
Other		cephazolin	0.9
digoxin	0.8		
allopurinol* (oxypurinol)	0.8	*H_2-Antagonists*	
lithium	1.0	cimetidine	0.7
vancomycin	0.9	ranitidine	0.7
metformin	0.9	famotidine	0.7
vigabatrin	0.6		
		Other	
		aciclovir	0.7
		amantadine	0.9
		baclofen	0.8
		dalteparin	0.7
		fluconazole	0.8
		pethidine (norpethidine)	0.9

* metabolite with high fu; ** less with higher doses.

Dosing in the Elderly

Physiological function declines with age

More than 90% of the elderly population
(>65 yrs) receive prescription medicines and
it is estimated that 30% of these patients
suffer from adverse drug reactions (cf. 10%
of patients aged 20–30 years).

Elderly patients are not the same as the
younger population in their response to and
handling of drugs. Pharmacokinetics and
pharmacodynamics may both be altered in
the elderly patient.

Pharmacokinetics

Clearance (Cl): this is by far the most important parameter with respect to dosing. Both
renal and liver clearance decline with age.

Renally eliminated drugs (i.e. large fu)

Drug Cl of drugs with high fu is
consistently impaired in the elderly

The principles outlined in 'Dosing in Renal
Impairment', see page 30, apply. The elderly
patient may have a 'normal' serum creatinine
[Cr] but the CrCl may be considerably impaired. This is because [Cr] is a reflection
of both production (from muscles) and elimination through the kidneys. Production
of creatinine is considerably lower in the
elderly than in fit young adults. The Cockcroft & Gault equation adjusts for age and
weight to allow for the decrease in creatinine
production.

$$CrCl(mL/s) = \frac{(140-age) \times wt[kg]}{50\,000 \times [Cr](mmol/L)}$$

× 0.85 (in females because of a higher ratio
of fat to lean body weight).

The dose-rate (DR) is then calculated as in
renal impairment:
For drugs with fu close to 1

$$\frac{DR(patient)}{DR(normal)} = \frac{calculated\ CrCl}{1.5}$$

For drugs with fu >0.5 but <1

$$\frac{DR(patient)}{DR(normal)} = (1 - fu) + fu \times \left(\frac{calculated\ CrCl}{1.5} \right)$$

As always this is especially important for
drugs with a low therapeutic index.

Metabolized drugs

Drug Cl of metabolized drugs is
usually impaired in the elderly

There is increasing evidence of impaired
metabolism of drugs in the elderly, though
this is less well defined compared with
renally eliminated drugs.

Perhaps the best advice is 'start low, go
slow'. Practically, this means beginning with
the lower end of the recommended dose
rates, and adjusting doses carefully thereafter. Dose intervals for drugs with short
half-lives can often be longer in the elderly.
Choose once or twice daily dosing where
possible to assist compliance.

Volume of distribution (Vd): The elderly
have decreased lean body mass, decreased
body water, and increased body fat compared with younger counterparts. Loading
doses of water-soluble drugs (smaller Vd)
should be based on ideal body weight, while
loading doses of fat-soluble drugs (larger
Vd) should be based on total body weight.

The half-life $(t_{1/2})$: The $t_{1/2}$ is often prolonged in the elderly. Longer $t_{1/2}$ means that the time to steady-state is longer, drug elimination takes longer, and dose-intervals may be longer. Often a longer half-life can be used to advantage if it allows for a once daily or twice daily regimen instead of three or four times daily.

Pharmacodynamics

Homeostatic adaptation is less efficient and target organ sensitivity may be altered in the elderly.

Homeostatic responses tend to be blunted, e.g. orthostatic hypotension is more pronounced in elderly patients due to a reduced ability of the baroreceptors to compensate for changes in blood pressure.

Target organ sensitivity is often altered (usually blunted). Alterations in receptor function may occur with age, e.g. impairment of cholinergic and adrenergic function.

Enhancing compliance
(see Compliance with Medication, page 76)

It is especially useful in the elderly to follow all the rules for enhancing compliance. Economy in the use of drugs, single-dose regimens, once or twice daily dosing, clear instructions and the use of compliance aids can enhance therapeutics markedly. Compliance aids include cards listing all the drugs and their dosing regimens, patient information leaflets and unit dose packaging.

General guidelines
1 Consider dosing reduction in patients over 55 yrs
2 Use estimate of CrCl to adjust dose of drugs with high fu
3 Start low, go slow for metabolized drugs
4 Aim for twice or once daily dosing
5 Monitor more frequently, especially for drugs with a low therapeutic index
6 Use as few drugs as possible
7 Provide a card listing the patient's drugs and dose regimen
8 Give patient information leaflets if available
9 Consider unit dose packaging

Dosing in Children

A child is not a little adult

2

The seven ages of pharmacological man	
Premature neonate	24/40–40/40
Neonate	0–2/12
Infant	2/12–1 year
Child	1–12 years
Adolescent	12–20 years
Adult	20–65 years
Aged	>65 years

Approximate values of Cl at different ages.

Post-conceptual age	Cl (cf adults)
24–28 weeks	5%
28–34 weeks	10%
34–40 weeks	33%
40–44 weeks	50%
44–68 weeks	66%
>68 weeks	100%

There are seven distinct age groups that are associated with different drug Cl and hence dosing requirements. Note that four of these ages are related to the paediatric age group. This reflects that the child is a continually changing pharmacokinetic and pharmacodynamic environment. The younger the child, the greater the rate of change.

Dosing in children under 6 months of age is very complicated — specialist advice is usually needed.

Pharmacokinetics

Clearance (Cl): The major mechanisms of drug elimination begin to develop during fetal life and continue to develop postpartum. Functional maturity is reached between 6 months and 1 year of age. After this, Cl is actually greater than that of adults on a mg/kg basis. It then relates better to surface area.

The major metabolic pathways, p450 oxidation and glucuronidation, and the renal pathways, all mature at a similar rate and can be considered together in their effects on drug Cl and dosage.

e.g. theophylline   (p450 oxidation)
      chloramphenicol (glucuronidation)
      gentamicin   (glomerular filtration)
These are all impaired in the neonate.

Volume of distribution (Vd): The infant has more body water and less fat than an adult as a percentage of total weight, i.e. up to 85% water in the premature neonate (cf 60% in an adult). The Vd is therefore increased for water soluble drugs and decreased for lipid soluble drugs. However, these effects are small compared with the changes in Cl in this age group, and dose-adjustment, if any, is small.

Protein binding (PB): PB is decreased in neonates due to decreased albumin, decreased binding capacity and the presence of displacers such as free fatty acids and bilirubin. However, this has little significance apart from in the interpretation of drug concentrations (see Protein Binding, page 14).

Drug availability: The **extent** of oral availability is not altered significantly. Skin absorption of some compounds may be enhanced because of a thinner stratum corneum, and a higher degree of hydration of the skin. Drugs should be applied sparingly.

Pharmacodynamics

Paediatric patients may be more sensitive to the effects of some drugs, e.g. aspirin toxicity. The blood–brain barrier is slow to develop enabling enhanced CNS effects with some drugs, e.g. increased transport of bilirubin into the brain may result in kernicterus. There may be paradoxical reactions, e.g. stimulation with benzodiazepines; control of hyperactivity with amphetamines.

Dosing guidelines

Under 6 months

Specialist advice necessary.

6 months–12 years

Use surface area (SA) approach
1 Using nomograms:
   Read SA from a nomogram

$$\text{Maintenance dose} = \frac{SA[m^2]}{1.73 \ m^2} \times \text{adult dose}$$

2 Without nomograms:
  A useful guide is:

Body weight (kg)	SA
10	0.5
20	0.75
30	1.0
40	1.25

Interpolate and extrapolate as necessary and use in above equation.
3 Using a calculator:
  In the absence of an estimate of surface area, an adjusted body weight can be used as follows:

$$\text{Maintenance dose} = \frac{Wt[kg]^{0.7}}{70} \times \text{adult dose}$$

This equation is derived from the fact that weight to the power of 0.7 ($wt^{0.7}$) relates better to surface area than to weight alone.

Drugs in Pregnancy

2

All drugs pass across the placenta to some extent, and therefore some fetal exposure will occur

Up to 95% of women take four or more drugs (not counting vitamin supplements) at some stage during pregnancy.

There are two major considerations regarding drugs in pregnancy.
1 The effects that the drugs have on the pregnancy.
2 The effects that the pregnancy has on the drugs.

Effects of drugs on the pregnancy

The majority of drugs attain concentrations in the fetus similar to those of maternal plasma.

It is important to remember that approximately 3–5% of all live births are associated with a fetal abnormality. Drugs are thought to be responsible for only 1–5% of these (i.e. 0.03–0.25% of all malformations). Association does not necessarily imply causation.

Exposure during the first 16 weeks of pregnancy is associated with an increased incidence of physical malformations. However, less obvious effects such as decreased neuronal function or impaired intellectual development may occur following exposure at any time during pregnancy.

(a) **Teratogenicity:** This is difficult to predict prior to marketing. Information comes from retrospective studies and/or animal data (often unreliable). The FDA classify drugs (see below), in increasing order of potential toxicity.

(b) **Pharmacological risks:** These are risks that are generally predictable based on the known pharmacology of the drug, e.g. NSAIDs may cause premature closure of the ductus arteriosus in the latter stages of pregnancy (patency requires the presence of prostaglandins).

At term, excessive effects (e.g. tricyclics) and withdrawal syndromes (e.g. opiates, selective serotonin reuptake inhibitors [SSRIs]) may be seen in neonates following maternal use.

Effects of pregnancy on drugs

Clearance (Cl): Pregnancy is generally a hyperdynamic physiological state. Drug clearance may be increased, whether it be via renal elimination or liver metabolism. The maternal cardiac output is increased by up to 30% during pregnancy, increasing the renal blood flow and GFR. The hormonal state in pregnancy is also associated with enzyme induction of some drugs. Maintenance doses of drugs often need to be

---

- **Category A** — Controlled studies in animals and women have not shown risk.
- **Category B** — Animal studies have not shown risk but there are no controlled studies in pregnant women **or** animal studies have shown risk but controlled studies in women have not. (e.g. paracetamol, β-lactams, methyldopa, NSAIDs [NSAIDs not safe in 3rd trimester]).
- **Category C** — Animal studies have shown risk but studies in women have not done so. (e.g. antipsychotics, most cardiac medicines, laxatives, antihistamines).
- **Category D** — Positive evidence of some human risk exists but benefits may in some circumstances outweigh risk. (e.g. anticonvulsants, ethanol, warfarin, antidepressants, tetracyclines, diuretics, lithium).
- **Category X** — Too dangerous — contraindicated. (e.g. thalidomide, vitamin A analogues, some cytotoxics).

Drugs associated with teratogenicity.

Drug	Outcome
Alcohol	Fetal alcohol syndrome
Anticonvulsants	
carbamazepine	Fetal carbamazepine syndrome
	• similar to fetal hydantoin syndrome
	• microcephaly, short nose
phenobarbitone	Similar to fetal hydantoin syndrome
phenytoin	Fetal hydantoin syndrome
	• impaired growth, craniofacial defects, mental deficiency, hypoplastic phalanges/nails
sodium valproate	Neural tube defects
Antithyroid drugs	Goitre, hypothyroidism
Cytotoxics	Multiple abnormalities, especially craniofacial/skeletal
Diethylstilboestrol	Masculinized genitalia
	Vaginal adhesions/carcinoma
Lithium	Ebstein's anomaly (structural cardiac deformity)
Penicillamine	Skin hyperelasticity
Tetracyclines	Tooth staining in offspring
Thalidomide	Phocomelia (limb reduction defects)
Vitamin A derivatives	
retinoic acid	Spontaneous abortion
tretinoin	Craniofacial abnormalities
etretinate	
Warfarin	Fetal warfarin syndrome
	• skeletal abnormalities
	• hypoplastic nose

increased during pregnancy, to compensate for increased Cl.

Volume of distribution (Vd): Vd may be increased by ~20% for both lipid- and water-soluble drugs. Increased loading doses may be required because of an increase in both body fat and water.

Protein binding (PB) [see page 14]: Maternal albumin concentrations decrease throughout pregnancy to a low at term. Measured drug concentrations of highly protein-bound drugs (e.g. phenytoin) may be lower, but this is usually unimportant, as free concentrations are not affected (see Protein Binding, page 14). Assessment requires specialist advice.

> The risk/benefit ratio must be considered when drugs are used in pregnancy

General advice

1 Avoid **all** drugs if possible, including social drugs (e.g. smoking, alcohol, caffeine)
2 Avoid drugs in the first trimester
3 Choose drugs of proven safety or least toxicity
4 Use short courses and the smallest doses.

Drugs in Human Milk

> All drugs diffuse into breast milk to some extent — it is the extent that is important

> Infant exposure to drugs during breast feeding is almost always less than exposure during pregnancy

> The infant derives no benefit from the drug — an innocent bystander

Most drugs pass into milk by **passive diffusion** of the free (unbound) and unionized form. They are distributed within the aqueous, protein and lipid phases of milk. Milk contains more fat and less protein than blood. Therefore drugs that are highly lipid soluble, with low protein binding, and unionized at physiological pH achieve higher concentrations in milk. Few drugs have concentrations in milk higher than those of maternal plasma.

The risk to the infant of medicine ingested via maternal milk may be considered from three viewpoints.
1 The 'dose' of medicine ingested by the infant.
2 The resulting infant plasma concentration.
3 The potential toxicity of that concentration.

The dose ingested by the infant

The most commonly used index that enables the dose to be calculated is the **milk/plasma ratio** (M/P). The most valid M/P ratio is that based on the AUC of drug in milk compared with the AUC in maternal plasma (i.e. M/P_{AUC}). The M/P ratio enables the concentration of the drug in milk to be estimated from knowledge of the maternal plasma concentration (C_{mat}).

The infant dose can be estimated from the maternal plasma concentration, the M/P ratio and the volume of milk (V_{milk}) ingested (150 mL/kg/day).

$$\text{Dose}_{infant} = C_{mat} * M/P * V_{milk}$$

A better index of dose is the actual amount of drug present in the milk over the maternal dosage interval.

The infant dose can be put into clinical perspective by comparison with the maternal dose (mg/kg), or with doses used therapeutically in the infant.

The weight-adjusted maternal dose (WAMD) is the dose the infant receives via milk, compared with the mother's dose, corrected for respective weights. It is usually expressed as a percentage, which if <10% (for a relatively non-toxic drug) indicates that the drug may be considered compatible with breast feeding.

The infant plasma concentration (C_{infant})

This depends on the dose-rate, the oral availability (F) and the drug clearance in the infant.

$$C_{infant} = \frac{\text{dose-rate} * F}{Cl}$$

F is usually assumed to be equivalent to that of adults, although this may not be so. Drug clearance is considerably impaired in infants less than 3 months of age, and especially so in the premature neonate. Thus an apparently small 'dose' may result in clinically significant plasma concentrations in the infant. Approximate values of Cl at different ages that enable calculation of appropriate concentrations in infants are shown below.

Post-conceptual age	CI (cf adults)
24–28 weeks	5%
28–34 weeks	10%
34–40 weeks	33%
40–44 weeks	50%
44–68 weeks	66%
>68 weeks	100%

wise even if the likely concentration in the infant is low. For other drugs, an arbitrary decision has to be made as to 'safe' concentrations in the infant. Predicted infant plasma concentrations of 10% of maternal concentrations are a useful cut-off point.

The potential toxicity of the drug in the infant

Breast-feeding during maternal ingestion of even small amounts of some very toxic drugs (e.g. antineoplastic drugs), is probably not

General advice regarding drugs in milk
1 Avoid drugs if possible
2 Weigh up the risk/benefit ratio
3 Exercise more caution with toxic agents
4 Feed baby just prior to the next dose
5 Alternate breast feeding with bottle feeding to decrease possible exposure

Drugs considered to be 'safe' when breast-feeding full-term healthy babies. (This table is a guide only, consult experts readily.)

Drug classes	Individual drugs	
ACE inhibitors	aciclovir	mebendazole
Antihistamines	5-aminosalicylic acid	methadone
Benzodiazepines	carbamazepine	methyldopa
β-lactam antibiotics	chlorothiazide	metoprolol
Calcium antagonists	citalopram	moclobemide
Oral contraceptives	clarithromycin	morphine
NSAIDs (except piroxicam)	codeine	nefopam
Phenothiazines	cotrimoxazole	nitrofurantoin
Tricyclic antidepressants	digoxin	paracetamol
	domperidone	paroxetine
	erythromycin	phenytoin
	famotidine	propranolol
	heparin	trimethoprim
	insulin	valproic acid
	labetalol	warfarin
	lignocaine	

Drugs considered to be 'unsafe' during breast-
feeding.

Amiodarone
Antineoplastic drugs
Ergotamine
Fluoroquinolones
Immunosuppressants
Iodine-containing agents
lithium
Retinoids
Tetracyclines
Social drugs, e.g. alcohol, cannabis,
Illegal drugs

---

3 Altered drug effect

3

Adverse Drug Reactions

An ADR is any response to a drug which is noxious, unintended, and occurs at doses used in man for prophylaxis, diagnosis or therapy.
WHO, 1976

Adverse drug reactions (ADRs) are a significant cause of morbidity and mortality and are responsible for around 5% of hospital admissions. Patients predisposed to ADRs are the elderly, females, and those with multiple disease, taking other drugs, and with a history of previous adverse reactions.

Classification

Type A (Augmented)	Type B (Bizarre)
Predictable	Unpredictable
Dose-dependent	Dose-independent
High incidence	Low incidence
(90% ADRs)	Often serious
May respond to	Generally need
dose adjustment	to stop drug

Type A (Augmented)

These reactions are predictable from the known pharmacology of the drug. They may result from an excessive *desired* response (e.g. hypotension from an antihypertensive) or non-specificity (e.g. anticholinergic effects with tricyclic antidepressants).

Pharmacokinetic mechanisms: Any patient with higher plasma concentrations than usual, due to inappropriate dosage or impaired clearance, is liable to type A adverse reactions. Examples are:
• renal dysfunction — aminoglycoside nephro/ototoxicity
• hepatic failure — prolonged sedation with benzodiazepines
• slow acetylator — isoniazid peripheral neuropathy
• slow hydroxylator — perhexiline peripheral neuropathy
• saturable kinetics — phenytoin ataxia
• drug interactions — erythromycin/terfenadine *torsades de pointes.*

Pharmacodynamic mechanisms: Some patients experience a type A ADR at a normal concentration, while others do not, reflecting natural variability. Similarly, underlying disease may shift the concentration–response curve to favour an ADR at a normal concentration, e.g. sedation in hepatic encephalopathy.

Prevention

• Take a careful history for predisposing factors.
• Use as small a dose as possible commensurate with desired effect.
• Adjust dosage to therapeutic end-points, e.g. BP or INR.
• Adjust dosage to optimum plasma concentrations, e.g. digoxin.
• Adjust dosage in relation to renal function, hepatic function, other disease states, or other drugs.

Management

• Decrease dose
• Substitute drug with different pharmacokinetics (e.g. metoprolol (metabolized) by atenolol (renally cleared))
• Consider alternative route of administration (e.g. transdermal vs oral)
• Substitute a more specific agent (e.g. moclobemide for tranylcypromine)
• Add drugs (carefully) to antagonize unwanted effects (e.g. addition of decarboxylase inhibitor to levodopa therapy (e.g. Sinemet, Madopar)

• Add another drug to allow reduced dose (e.g. diuretics + β-blockers).

Type B (Bizarre)

These are less common, less predictable, may be severe and result from various mechanisms. Examples are:
• immunologic — penicillin allergy
• pseudoallergy — asthma with NSAIDs
• genetic — haemolysis in G6PD deficiency
• disease — amoxycillin rash in glandular fever
• idiosyncratic — malignant hyperpyrexia in anaesthesia.

Prevention

• Take a careful drug history, especially of allergies
• Family history — allergies and genetic disease
• Avoid drugs susceptible to ADRs in particular disease states, e.g. clozapine in bone marrow depression.

Management

• **Stop drug** and treat symptomatically
• Avoid drugs with chemically similar groups, e.g. sulphonylureas and thiazide diuretics

• Do not rechallenge
• Notify CARM (Centre for Adverse Reaction Monitoring)
• Consider a Medic-Alert bracelet.

Assessing an ADR

The probability increases if the reaction:
• is appropriate to timing of drug administration
• follows a recognized pattern of response
• disappears on withdrawal of the drug
• reappears on rechallenge with drug
• responds appropriately to a specific antidote
• has happened before with the same or like drug
• is supported by measured toxic concentrations
• cannot be explained otherwise.

Reporting an ADR (to centre of adverse reactions)

The following information is needed:
• Case identification and patient data
• Description of ADR and its outcome
• Patient's diagnosis
• Concomitant drugs
• Predisposing/contributing factors
• Estimation of probability of drug causing the ADR
• The reporting doctor/pharmacist.

3

Drug-Induced Allergy

> Drug allergy is an adverse reaction, type B, mediated by an immunological mechanism

Drug-induced allergy results from previous sensitization to a particular chemical, or one that is structurally similar. The term 'hypersensitivity' is sometimes used for 'allergy' but has a broader meaning. Drug allergy is under-recognized, under-reported and probably represents about 20% of ADRs.

Most drugs have small molecular weights (often ~300 D) and are too small to be antigenic in themselves. They act as 'haptens', binding to endogenous proteins to form antigenic complexes that incite antibody production. This process usually takes 1–2 weeks. Reexposure to the chemical results in an antigen–antibody interaction that provokes the typical manifestations of allergy — release of mediators (e.g. histamine) cell damage or cell death.

Types of allergic reactions

Type I (immediate, anaphylactic)

Mediated by IgE and involves release of histamine, leukotrienes and prostaglandins causing vasodilation, oedema and a generalized inflammatory response (e.g. anaphylaxis, urticaria and bronchospasm due to penicillin).

Type II (cytotoxic)

Mediated by IgG and IgM through complement activation. The major targets are cells in the circulatory system (e.g. penicillin haemolytic anaemia, quinidine thrombocytopenia, sulphonamide neutropenia).

Type III (immune complex)

Mediated by IgG immune complexes and complement. The immune complexes block small blood vessels and cause a local inflammatory response. Serum sickness (urticaria, arthralgia, lymphadenopathy and fever), is a classical presentation (e.g. serum sickness due to sulphonamides or penicillins).

Extreme form — Stevens–Johnson syndrome.

Type IV (cell mediated)

Mediated by T-lymphocytes and macrophages. Sensitized cells release cytokines on contact with antigen (e.g. contact dermatitis by poison ivy).

Drug-induced autoimmune disease

This is not conveniently classifiable into the above. The drug alters a protein in the body so that the protein is no longer recognized as 'self' (e.g. drug-induced SLE).

Pseudoallergic reactions (anaphylactoid)

These are sometimes indistinguishable clinically from type I reactions. They are, however, mediated pharmacologically and not immunologically (e.g. aspirin and NSAIDs in asthma). The fact that they do not occur in everyone indicates some predisposition (e.g. genetic). This is why this type of reaction is considered to be type B rather than type A. Cross-sensitivity occurs with drugs which have the same action, but not structure, cf. true allergy.

Important points about drug-induced allergy

• May be due to the drug itself, a metabolite, or an excipient in the formulation.
• Usually highly specific to a chemical, but there may be cross-reactivity within a drug class, e.g. penicillins ~50% chance.
• The probability of cross-reactivity with chemically unrelated drugs is low.
• Patients with atopy may be predisposed to type I reactions.
• Many patients develop antibodies to drugs, but only a few develop clinically evident allergy.
• There is no correlation with known pharmacological properties of the drug.
• There is no consistent relationship with drug dose (although severity varies with dose).
• Usually resolves on cessation of drug.
• Reappears on rechallenge (often worse).
• Short-term desensitization is sometimes possible.
• It is unclear how long allergy may last, ?life-long, ?10–20 years.
• Assessment as for ADRs (page 42).

Percutaneous testing

Skin testing is theoretically attractive but has problems:
• May cause a severe reaction.
• **False positives**: Some drugs cause skin irritation, resembling wheal and flare (e.g. morphine). Others may sensitize topically without a systemic reaction (e.g. muscle relaxants).
• **False negatives**: Some drugs may not react topically, while producing a reaction systemically, e.g. allergy due to the metabolite rather than the drug (e.g. penicillin).

Prevention

• Avoid the use of drugs where cross-sensitivity is likely, especially if previous reaction to a chemically similar drug was severe.
• Use a small test dose.
• Have treatment ready, e.g. adrenaline, antihistamine, steroids.

For example, if a patient about to be treated reports an allergy to penicillin, it is important to determine what reaction actually occurred (e.g. mild rash versus anaphylaxis), and how long ago it happened. This will help decide whether a penicillin or other β-lactam (e.g. cephalosporin) could be used if they are drugs of choice for the condition. If the previous reaction was anaphylaxis, then both penicillins and cephalosporins (reported 5–10% cross-sensitivity) would be contraindicated. If, however, the previous reaction was minor, then a cephalosporin, or even a penicillin, might be considered reasonable. Of course in these circumstances a small test dose should be used, and treatment (e.g. adrenaline) should be readily available.

3

Adverse Drug Events

An adverse drug event (ADE) is actual or potential damage resulting from medical intervention related to medicines

Terminology is a problem here, because of confusion with adverse drug reactions (ADR) (see page 42). Other terms such as 'medication error' have been used but adverse drug event (ADE) seems to have been adopted the most widely. ADE covers a wider spectrum than adverse drug reaction and involves doctors, pharmacists, nurses, caregivers and patients themselves. Omitting a dose is an ADE, while a rash is an ADR.

What comprises an ADE?

Prescribing error:
- incorrect drug selection
- incorrect dose or frequency
- incorrect route of administration
- inappropriate duration of therapy
- incorrect prescription
- incomplete prescription
- illegible prescription
- unforeseen drug interaction.

Medication error:
- transcription error
- dispensing error
- infusion error
- failure to uplift prescription
- non-compliance
- inadequate monitoring.

Why are ADEs important?

ADEs are common and result in significant morbidity and mortality. Alarming statistics from the US, UK and Australia suggest that ADEs may be one of the leading causes of death (behind heart disease, cancer and stroke). The cost of this is huge and the incid-ence is increasing. More important, however, is that most of these are **preventable**.

Why do ADEs occur?

'ADEs are primarily a result of system problems, not people problems'.

Dr Lucian Leape, Harvard School of Public Health

On the surface ADEs appear to be the result of human error. However human error abounds when systems predispose.

Major systems failures: (from *JAMA*, 1995; 274: 35–43). The following are responsible for over 70% of errors:
- Lack of knowledge about drugs e.g. failure to recognize that a drug is renally cleared.
- Lack of information about patient e.g. failure to recognize that a patient has renal failure.
- Violation of rules: e.g. incomplete prescription such as route not stated.
- Slips and memory lapses e.g. doctor forgets to prescribe post-op analgesia.
- Transcription errors e.g. wrong dose.
- Faulty drug identification e.g. moclobemide for metoclopramide.

Preventing errors

Efforts that focus on the individual who made the error ('shoot the messenger') are usually unfruitful. The essence is to alter systems to minimize the chance of errors occurring. Each of the above system failures should be addressed.
- Drug knowledge: Information about all aspects of the drug profile must be readily available at the time the drug is prescribed/used.

• Patient information: Clinical information, results of laboratory tests, drug history and allergies, current medications and doses must be accessible and known at the time of using the drug.

• Following the rules: Poor prescribing should not be tolerated and 'covered for' by pharmacists. Quality assurance programs with feedback can assist. See Preventing Adverse Drug Events, page 48.

• Slips and memory lapses: Excessive workloads should be avoided. Quality assurance programs with 'no blame' should be encouraged.

• Transcription errors: Single point of data entry should be encouraged.

• Drug identity: Avoid illegibility e.g. UPPER CASE letters for drug names.

A computerized prescribing system linked to drug and patient information databases could fix many of the above problems. Unfortunately, this requires quite a commitment both financially and from top-level management. It is also complex to develop.

Preventing Adverse Drug Events

An ADE is any event (or potential event) that occurs as a result of an error in any part of the process of drug administration

Examples of medication errors that have caused death

• Wrong drug: frusemide instead of flutamide. *Outcome* — death from acute renal failure.
• Wrong dose: mg instead of mcg. *Outcome* — death from overdose.
• Wrong route: vincristine into intrathecal space. *Outcome* — death from neurotoxicity.
• Wrong instructions: chronic lorazepam withdrawn over 3 days instead of 3 weeks. *Outcome* — rebound panic/anxiety causing suicide.

Some reasons for medication errors

• Prescriber:
Poor knowledge about patient (e.g. history of allergy, serum creatinine);
Poor knowledge of drug, e.g. cleared renally, but dose not adjusted;
Missed drug interactions;
Poor prescription: illegible, incomplete, prescriber unidentifiable.
• Pharmacist:
Mis-reading prescription;
Transcribing error;
Dispensing error.
• Nurse:
Drug given to wrong patient;
Wrong drug given;
Wrong dose given.
• Patient:
Failure to uplift prescription;
Non-compliance.
• Adverse prescribing culture:
Understaffing;
False economies;
Poor communication;
Tolerance of laxity.
• Modern drug therapy:
increasing complexity;
multiple medications;
drug interactions.

Examples of common errors in prescribing (all aggravated by illegibility).

qd (once daily) confused with qid (4 times daily)	use qid
IU (international units) confused with IV (intravenous)	write 'I units'
U (units) confused with 0 (zero)	write 'units'
pm (afternoon or night) confused with prn (as required)	use nocte
2.0 mg (2 mg) confused with 20 mg	write 2 mg
.5 mg (half a mg) confused with 5 mg	write 0.5 mg
µg (microgram) confused with mg (milligram)	write mcg
< or > (less or greater than) confused with 4 or 7	write in full

How to avoid errors

- Acknowledge the problem:
  Allow for human nature;
  Non-punitive reporting system.
- Cooperative approach between:
  doctor/pharmacist/nurse.
- Encourage favourable behaviour patterns.
- Computerized prescribing system.

Risk reduction strategies

(see Patients and their drugs, page 80)
- Prescriptions:
  Avoid abbreviations where possible (write in full);
  Only use acceptable, non-ambiguous abbreviations;
  Write clearly;
  Provide adequate detail (specific instructions);
  Use UPPER CASE letters for drug names;
  Write prescriber's name in UPPER CASE alongside signature;
  Do not alter a prescription — rewrite it;
  Take particular care with decimal points.

- Encouraging compliance:
  Medication card;
  Patient Information leaflets;
  Unit dose packaging devices.

Acceptable abbreviations

bd — Twice daily
tds — Three times daily
qid — Four times daily
qXh — Every X hours
mane — in the morning
nocte — at night
prn — As required
ac — Before food
pc — After food
im — Intramuscular
iv — Intravenous
po — Oral
pr — Rectal
sc — Subcutaneous

3

If ambiguity is possible in a prescription, write the details out in full

Drug/Drug Interactions

> A drug interaction occurs when the effects of one drug are increased or decreased by the previous or concurrent administration of another

- Patients on six or more drugs have an 80% chance of a drug interaction. (*NB*: hospital in-patients receive, on average, around six drugs at any one time).
- Consequence of a drug interaction is that dose alteration may be necessary, or alternative medications prescribed.
- Interactions are most important for drugs with a low therapeutic index.
- The sicker the patient, the greater the risk of a drug interaction.
- Not all interactions are bad.

> **Mechanisms**
> - Pharmacokinetic
> - Pharmacodynamic
> - Pharmaceutic

Pharmacokinetic

A change in blood concentration occurs causing a change in effect.

Altered availability

- Chelation within the gut
  e.g. tetracyclines/Ca^{2+} → ↓ [tetracycline]
- Altered motility
  e.g. metoclopramide/digoxin → ↓ [digoxin]
- Altered first-pass metabolism
  e.g. oestrogens/ascorbic acid → ↑ [oestrogen]
- Altered bacterial flora
  e.g. antibiotics/sulphasalazine → ↓ cleavage of sulphasalazine in large intestine.

Altered elimination

Interactions may occur at metabolic or renal sites of elimination. Metabolic interactions include enzyme induction or inhibition. These happen especially with drugs metabolized by cytochrome-P450-mediated metabolism.

Enzyme induction

Strong enzyme inducers affect many drugs and include:
- anticonvulsants (phenytoin, carbamazepine)
- rifampicin
- smoking and alcoholism.

Enzyme induction involves increased synthesis of the enzyme involved. Most types of metabolism are inducible, although there are notable exceptions, e.g. CYP2D6. The effect of enzyme induction is to increase first-pass metabolism, increase clearance, decrease $t_{1/2}$ and lower average steady-state concentrations.

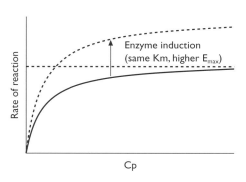

Enzyme inhibition

Strong enzyme inhibitors affect many drugs and include:
- erythromycin
- selective serotonin reuptake inhibitors (SSRIs)

50

- ketoconazole
- amiodarone
- cimetidine
- grapefruit juice.

Enzyme inhibition causes less first-pass metabolism, decreased clearance, longer $t_{1/2}$ and higher average steady-state concentrations.

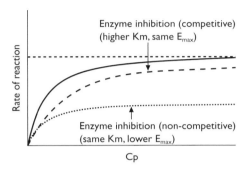

All types of drug metabolism may be affected by enzyme inhibition. Some inhibitions are so profound that the average steady-state concentrations increase greater than 10-fold, e.g. grapefruit juice increases lovastatin concentrations by up to 16-fold through inhibition of CYP3A4 first-pass metabolism.

Renal excretion

- Altered pH of urine
  e.g. HCO_3^- → ↑ aspirin excretion

- Competition for active secretion in proximal tubule
  e.g. probenecid/penicillin → ↑ [penicillin]
- Competition for ionic cotransport
  e.g. Li^+/Na^+ → Li^+ accumulation with diuretics.

Pharmacodynamic

Drug effect is altered through receptor, cellular or other physiological mechanisms. Enhancement or antagonism may occur.
e.g. β-agonist/β-blocker-mutual competition at receptor site.

Pharmaceutic

Physicochemical interactions may occur 'prior' to systematic availability
e.g. inactivation of phenytoin within IV giving sets if pH is <7.0.

Practical notes

1 Take *full* drug history, including asking about over-the-counter (OTC) preparations.
2 Interactions are likely with more than three concurrent drugs.
3 Use as few drugs, for as short a time, as possible.
4 Monitor effect or Cp assiduously.
5 Review all medication frequently.
6 Pharmacodynamic interactions are likely to be shared within same drug class.

Some drug classes and drugs with important interactions	
• antiarrhythmics — cause enzyme inhibition	• cyclosporin
• anticonvulsants — cause enzyme induction	• digoxin
• anticoagulants — multiple mechanisms	• hypoglycaemic agents
• antidepressants — cause enzyme inhibition	• lithium
• protease inhibitors — cause enzyme inhibition	• theophylline

Inducers of Drug Metabolism

Class	Drug	CYP enzyme affected
Anticonvulsants	phenobarbitone	3A4, 2C9, 2C19
	phenytoin	3A4, 2C9, 2C19
	carbamazepine	3A4, 2C19
Antibiotics	rifampicin	3A4, 2C9, 2C19, 1A2
	rifabutin	3A4
	griseofulvin	3A4, 2C9, 2C19
	sulphaphenazole	2C9
	isoniazid	2E1
Steroids	glucocorticoids	3A4
	progesterone	3A4
Social drugs	alcohol	2E1
	marijuana	1A2
	cigarettes	1A2
Foods	barbequed foods	1A2
	cruciferous vegetables (cabbage, broccoli, brussel sprouts, cauliflower)	1A2
Environmental toxins	cyclic hydrocarbons	1A2
	dioxane, DDT	1A2
Other	phenylbutazone	2C9
	omeprazole	1A2
	ritonavir	1A2
	efavirenz	3A4
	nevirapine	3A4
	barbiturates	3A4, 2C9, 2C19
	St John's Wort	3A4

Inhibitors of Drug Metabolism

Class	Drug	CYP enzyme affected
Microsomal		
Antiarrhythmics	amiodarone	1A, 2C9, 2D6, 3A4
	propafenone, quinidine	2D6
Antibiotics	chloramphenicol	2C9
	sulphonamides	2C9
	trimethoprim	2C9
	azole antifungals	1A2, 2C9, 2C19, 3A4
	macrolides	1A2, 3A4
	quinolones	1A2, 3A4
Antiulcer	cimetidine	1A2, 2C9, 2C19, 2D6, 3A4
	omeprazole	1A2, 2C9, 2C19, 3A4
	lansoprazole	2C19
Calcium antagonists	diltiazem	3A4, 2D6
	verapamil	3A4
Antidepressants	fluoxetine	2C19, 2D6, 3A4
	paroxetine	2D6
	moclobemide	2C19, 2D6
	nefazodone	3A4
Antipsychotics	chlorpromazine, fluphenazine	2D6
	haloperidol, thioridazine	2D6
Protease inhibitors	indinavir, saquinavir, nelfinavir	3A4
	ritonavir	2C9, 2D6, 3A4
Statins	fluvastatin, lovastatin	2C9
Other	isoniazid	2C9, 2C19, 3A4
	oral contraceptives	3A4
	metoprolol, propranolol	2D6
	sodium valproate	2C9, 2C19, 2D6, 3A4
	ticlopidine	1A2, 2C19
	methylphenidate	2C9, 2C19, 2D6
	dextropropoxyphere	3A4, 2D6, 2C9
	terbinafine	2D6
Extramicrosomal		
	disulfiram	aldehyde dehydrogenase, 2E1
	ascorbic acid	sulphation
	allopurinol	xanthine oxidase
	MAOIs	MAO

Drug/Food Interactions

Food may alter the pharmacokinetics
of a drug, and/or its action

Food and pharmacokinetics

Food may alter drug availability (absorption
and first-pass metabolism), drug distribution and drug clearance.

Absorption

Altered **rate** or **extent** of absorption may
occur. Altered RATE is of little importance unless immediate effect is required, e.g.
analgesics. Large, hot, fatty, solid meals
decrease, and fluid-based meals increase the
rate of absorption.

Food may decrease the **extent** of absorption, particularly of polar, hydrophilic, lipid
insoluble drugs, e.g. atenolol. Stimulation of
gastric enzymes and acid may degrade some
drugs, e.g. flucloxacillin.

Iron, calcium and other divalent or trival-
ent ions (e.g. dairy products or in supplements) may chelate some drugs decreasing
extent of absorption, e.g. quinolones and
tetracyclines are chelated by antacids, and
by calcium in milk.

First-pass metabolism

In general, food increases liver blood flow
from the gut causing increased **extent** of
availability of drugs subject to high first-pass
metabolism (see page 12). This happens because increased presentation of drug to the
hepatocytes saturates metabolic processes,
allowing more drug to get through to the circulation, e.g. metoprolol.

Grapefruit juice

A component(s) in grapefruit inhibits the
CYP3A4 enzymes responsible for metabolizing many drugs as they pass through the gut
wall. This may lead to large increases in serum
concentrations of susceptible drugs. Drugs
affected have the following characteristics:
- Metabolized largely by CYP3A4
- Subject to marked first-pass metabolism.

Increases in the AUC of up to 16-fold have
been reported, e.g. lovastatin.

Drugs affected by grapefruit juice	
• amlodipine	• lovastatin
• atorvastatin	• midazolam
• buspirone	• nifedipine
• carbamazepine	• nimodipine
• cisapride	• saquinavir
• cyclosporin	• simvastatin
• diltiazem	• tacrolimus
• ethinyloestradiol	• triazolam
• felodipine	• verapamil

Drug distribution

Altered drug distribution is not usually a
major problem because distribution is not
relevant to steady-state plasma concentrations. However, if distribution to a site of
drug activity is affected then it is important,
e.g. high protein diet decreases the uptake
of L-dopa into the CNS by competition
between amino acids and L-dopa at the
blood–brain barrier.

Drug clearance

Drug clearance may be enhanced by foods
associated with enzyme induction, e.g. high
protein meals, barbequed food, cruciferous
vegetables (broccoli and cabbage). This
mainly affects CYP1A2. In order for this to

be a problem, the diet must be constant, because enzyme induction takes 2–3 weeks to reach a new equilibrium.

Altered drug effects

Some foods contain substances that act on the same receptors or sites of action as drugs. Agonistic or antagonistic effects may be observed.
• Liquorice contains glycyrrhizic acid which is similar to aldosterone, and causes water retention, increased BP and antagonism of antihypertensive drugs.
• Foods high in vitamin K (beef liver, avocado, leafy green vegetables, egg yolk, broccoli, soybeans, chickpeas, lentils) may antagonize warfarin by competitive inhibition.
• Alcohol may cause sedation/respiratory depression with CNS depressants, e.g.

benzodiazepines, antidepressants, antipsychotics, opiates.

Effects of drugs on food

Drugs may alter the concentration or effect of substances in foods and drink. For example:
• Stimulant laxatives (senna, biscodyl) and diuretics may cause electrolyte losses.
• Orlistat and bile-acid sequestrants may decrease the absorption of fat-soluble vitamins (A, D, E, K).
• Enzyme inducers (rifampicin, anticonvulsants) may induce the metabolism of vitamin D and folate causing respective deficiencies.
• Metronidazole causes a disulfiram-like reaction with alcohol.
• MAOIs cause 'the cheese reaction' with tyramine-containing foods causing a hypertensive crisis.

3

4 Pharmacovigilance

4

Drug Development

The development of a new drug is complex and expensive. The cost, from molecule to market, has been estimated to be in excess of US$250 million. The process takes many years.

The Holy Grail in drug development is the 'magic bullet'. This describes the ideal drug that is assimilated into the body with total predictability, homes in on its target with great specificity, interacts with no other receptors (i.e. adverse effect receptors), has no drug interactions, and is then eliminated predictably. This is impossible, of course. As Isaac Newton once said, 'Every action has an equal and opposite reaction'.

Drug discovery

Historically, drugs were often discovered serendipitously, e.g. penicillin. Targeting of drugs followed, using *in vitro* models that suggested desired activities. More recently a drug is usually discovered by design, e.g. specific receptor antagonist.

Preclinical drug development

Once purified, or synthesized, the drug is subject to a series of preclinical studies in animals. These are designed to confirm the activity, to explore dose–response relationships, to characterize the pharmacokinetics, to explore dose–response relationships, and to observe toxicological effect including mutagenicity and carcinogenicity. In recent years, these processes have come under intense scrutiny in relation to animal ethics, and are only conducted under rigidly controlled conditions. Where possible, computer modelling is used to minimize animal involvement.

Attention to formulation and pharmaceutical stability occurs concurrently. Only about 1% of compounds are judged suitable to move on to clinical testing.

Clinical drug development

This involves testing the drug in humans. The ethics of this are particularly important, and the process is subject to important regulations such as the Declaration of Helsinki. This states that 'Concern for the interests of the subject must always prevail over the interests of science and society'.

There are three phases, although the exact margins between the phases are sometimes blurred:

Phase I: (first time in humans) — basic clinical pharmacology

These studies are designed to observe the spectrum of pharmacological effects produced by a range of doses (i.e. dose–response evaluation) and the pharmacokinetic behaviour of the drug. The aim is to find a 'safe' dose for more detailed evaluation. An initial search for metabolites that might be different from those in animals is also undertaken.

These are open (not blind) studies, usually in small numbers (10–100) of normal volunteers (though sometimes in patients if the drug is particularly toxic, such as an antineoplastic agent), starting with low doses (suggested from animal studies). The studies are well supervised, usually by a clinical pharmacologist, and have a good safety record.

Phase II: Clinical investigation

These studies are designed to establish therapeutic effectiveness in patient volunteers who are suffering from the condition the drug is meant to help. Side effects are also studied. These are generally controlled trials (vs placebo or active comparator) and blinded (single or double blind), but in small numbers (100–300 total) and of short duration. The aim is to get a signal that the drug actually works and warrants the move to full-sized, statistically significant, randomized controlled trials. The pharmacokinetics in the relevant patient group are also examined, and perhaps in other selected patients such as those with renal or hepatic dysfunction. These studies are conducted by clinical pharmacologists and clinical investigators who are specialized in the patient group under study.

Phase III: Therapeutic trials

These are large-scale, randomized, controlled (vs placebo or active comparator) clinical trials in the patient group for whom the drug is intended, designed to prove conclusively that the drug has the desired effect and is suitably safe. These studies are well designed statistically, with adequate power to demonstrate clinically significant effects. The total number of patients studied is usually 1000–3000. The studies are undertaken by suitably qualified clinical investigators. Adverse effects are also monitored to detect incidences of >1 in 100 or thereabouts.

Post-marketing surveillance (sometimes termed phase IV)

During clinical development insufficient patients have been studied to detect rare and perhaps serious adverse events. There are intensive monitoring schemes in most countries to detect such events. In addition, unexpected benefits in patient groups or diseases other than those initially targeted may be observed, and drug interactions detected.

Regulatory process

The same general process follows in most countries although the detail might differ.

IND — Investigational New Drug application

The preclinical (animal) evidence is evaluated in order to allow studies to proceed to phase I studies.

NDA — New Drug application

The clinical evidence (Phase I, II, and III) is evaluated for approval to allow the drug to be marketed.

Ethical considerations

At all stages of drug development (including animal studies) ethical approval is required before a study can proceed. General ethical guidelines were drawn up in 1947 under the Nurenburg Code. In 1964 the Declaration of Helsinki was adopted by the World Medical Association. This has been revised three times since then and remains the cornerstone of ethical principles behind drug studies.

The process, while clearly laudable and politically correct, has become increasingly stringent, and is in danger of actually preventing advancement. This must be guarded against.

4

Therapeutic Drug Monitoring (TDM)

TDM describes the monitoring of concentrations of drugs in body fluids, usually plasma, for therapeutic purposes

Why?

Therapeutic drug monitoring (TDM) helps (for relevant drugs) to increase *efficacy*, to decrease *toxicity*, and to assist *diagnosis*.

Theoretical basis and assumptions

For some drugs the relationship between dose and effect is so variable that the choice of dose regimen is difficult.

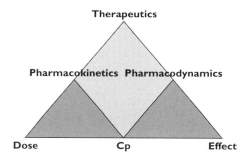

Measurement of plasma concentrations (Cp) gets us closer to the 'effect compartment'.
• Assumption — Equilibrium exists between plasma and tissue concentrations.
NB: When plasma concentrations are measured, the Cp refers to *total* drug in plasma, including protein bound drug, unless specifically stated:

Cp = bound drug + unbound drug

Indications for TDM

(a) Improvement in efficacy

'Prophylactic' drugs — some drugs such as antiarrhythmics and anticonvulsants are used to *prevent* undesired effects. Waiting for an end-point to occur such as ventricular tachycardia is too dangerous.

Drugs with pharmacokinetic problems — drugs with a poor dose–concentration relationship have a poor dose-effect relationship (e.g. phenytoin — non-linear kinetics).

Drug interactions or disease states (especially liver of renal dysfunction) may alter the dose–concentration relationship.

(b) Avoidance of toxicity

Drugs with a low 'therapeutic index' require individualized dosing.

(i) Low therapeutic index

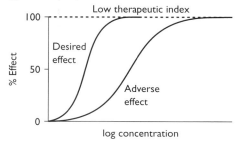

(ii) High therapeutic index

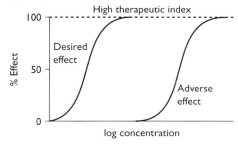

(c) Diagnosis

Failure of therapy: TDM helps distinguish between genuine drug resistance (inappropriate agent), non-compliance, and adverse effects that mimic the disease state.

Overdose: Cp measurement may distinguish drug-induced from organic disease (e.g. coma caused by sedative overdose). A decision to use an antidote can be assisted and prognosis assessed by using nomograms that relate Cp to likely toxicity, e.g. paracetamol.

Drug abuse: Confirmation of abstinence, e.g. narcotic treatment programmes, athletic screening.

For which drugs?

See page 62.

When to measure?

The timing of blood sampling and the last dose is critical and must be recorded.

A trough concentration (i.e. just prior to the next dose) is the usual measure of drug accumulation. Occasionally, sampling at the time of symptoms may detect 'peak' concentration toxicity.

Some drugs, e.g. gentamicin, may require measurement of two concentrations within the dosing interval, to assess peak and trough concentrations, or to calculate an AUC.

Steady-state concentrations (i.e. >4 half-lives after dose initiation or change in dose) are relevant to chronic therapy.

The 'therapeutic range'

This is the range of drug concentrations associated with a reasonable probability of **efficacy**, without undue **toxicity** in the majority of patients. In practice this 'range' is not well established for most drugs, and is a guide only.

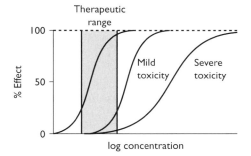

Problems with TDM

The illusion of scientific accuracy, the dubious validity of some therapeutic ranges, laboratory variation, active (unmeasured) metabolites, and failure of the basic assumptions all make the use of TDM difficult. Consult readily.

> Treat the patient, not the laboratory value

Drugs Involved in Therapeutic Drug Monitoring

Remember:
- therapeutic drug monitoring only **assists** clinical judgement
- most reference ranges refer to trough concentrations

- check units of measurement (mg/L vs μmol/L)
- consult readily.

Drugs that should be monitored 'routinely'.

Class	Reference range	Comment
Aminoglycosides		
Gentamicin	AUC 70–100 mg/L.h	How to monitor once daily aminoglycosides still debated
Tobramycin	Trough <0.5 mg/L	
Netilmicin	AUC 150–200 mg/L.h	
Amikacin		
Carbamazepine	16–48 μmol/L	Upper limit subject to debate
	4–12 mg/L	
Cyclosporin	Induction 100–300 μg/L	Different ranges quoted for different transplants
	Maintenance 100–200 μg/L	
Flucytosine	200–800 μmol/L	Bone marrow toxicity >800 mmol/L
	25–100 mg/L	
Lithium	Acute mania 0.8–1.2 mmol/L	
	Prophylaxis 0.4–0.8 mmol/L	
Phenytoin	40–80 μmol/L	Saturable kinetics
	10–20 mg/L	In hypoalbuminaemia measure free concentrations
	Free 4–8 μmol/L	

Drugs for which monitoring may be useful.

Class	Reference range	Comment
Amiodarone	1–4 µmol/L (parent), 0.5–2.5 mg/L	Very long $t_{1/2}$
Aspirin	Rheumatic fever 250–400 mg/L Overdose >400 mg/L	Saturable kinetics at higher doses
Carboplatin	AUC 80–120 mg/L.h AUC 50–80 mg/L.h	Ovarian/testicular cancer
Chloramphenicol	15–20 mg/L	Dose-related toxicity
Digoxin	1–2.5 nmol/L, 0.8–2 µg/L	Trough concentration or >8h post-dose
Flecainide	0.2–1 mg/L	Subject to slow CTP2D6 polymorphism
Isoniazid	1–7 mg/L, Toxic >20 mg/L	
Itraconazole	Trough >250 g/L	Monitor for efficacy
Lamotrigine	3–14 mg/L	Revised upwards from 1–4 mg/L
Lignocaine	1.5–5 mg/L, Toxic >9 mg/L	Toxic metabolite
Methadone	0.3–1.3 µmol/L 100–400 µg/L	Considerable variation
Methotrexate	Toxic >10^{-6} mmol/L at 48 h Rx leucovorin	Monitor during high-dose therapy
Paracetamol	Toxic >1 mmol/L, >150 mg/L	Treatment level for N-acetylcystein (NAC)
Perhexiline	0.54–2.16 µmol/L, 0.15–0.6 mg/L	Subject to CYP2D6 polymorphism
Phenobarbitone	65–130 µmol/L, 15–30 mg/L	Long $t_{1/2}$
Tacrolimus	5–20 g/L (whole blood) 0.5–2 µg/L (plasma)	
Teicoplanin	10–20 mg/L 20–30 mg/L for deep infection	
Theophylline	55–110 µmol/L, 10–20 mg/L	
Valproic acid	50–100 mg/L, 350–700 µmol/L	Poorly established
Vancomycin	Trough 5–10 mg/L	Value of peaks not well established

4

Overdose/Poisoning

> 'All substance are poisons . . . It is
> only the amount that distinguishes
> a poison from a remedy'.
>
> *Paracelsus*

Poisoning accounts for ~1% of all admissions. Of these, <1% of patients die, largely a tribute to supportive care.

> The first priority is to keep the patient alive

A   Airways
B   Breathing
C   Circulation

First aid, supportive measures and decontamination

- The most important early management.
- Maintain fluid and electrolyte balance.
- Support vital systems, especially kidneys.
- Provide good nursing care.
- For the unconscious patient, monitor carefully, clear airway and place in coma position. Use CPR if necessary.
- If poisoned by gas, remove from source.
- Useful early management may include oxygen, naloxone and glucose.
- If conscious, give oral fluid.

Corrosive, acids, alkalis:

- Rinse mouth.
- Get patient to drink copious fluids.
- Drench affected skin, eyes, mucus membranes with water.
- Do *not* induce vomiting.

Petroleum products:

- Biggest danger is **inhalation**.
- Do *not* induce vomiting.
- Give a cupful of milk initially.

Diagnosis (see page 66)

Circumstantial evidence — pills, bottles, needles.
Clinical features — skin colour, pupils, BP, convulsions.
Laboratory — gastric aspirate, vomitus, blood, urine.

Measurement of concentrations

This may be useful as a prognostic indication and for determining whether active treatment is indicated.

Drugs for which Cp measurement may be useful see page 66.

Decreasing exposure

(i) Prevention of absorption

Emesis — May have a place in pre-hospital ingestion of drug by children. Not appropriate for adult ingestion.

Gastric lavage — indicated in the unconscious within 4 hours of ingestion, or longer for salicylates and poisons that delay gastric emptying. Contraindicated if cough reflex absent and cuffed endotracheal tube cannot be inserted.

Oral absorbents — activated charcoal adsorbs drug preventing further absorption. There is debate about their true place.

(ii) Enhanced elimination

Appropriate in <5% of poisonings and should be undertaken only by the experienced.

pH-adjusted diuresis: Alkaline diuresis may be useful in a few selected cases, e.g. aspirin. Benefits of acid diuresis more controversial.

Drugs for which pH-adjusted diuresis may help
Alkaline diuresis (for acids)
Phenobarbitone
Salicylates
Acidic diuresis (for bases)
Amphetamines
Methadone
Mexiletine
Phencyclidine
Phenylpropanolamines (e.g. pseudoephedrine, ephedrine)
Quinidine

Continuous activated charcoal: Drugs that continue to enter the gut via enterohepatic circulation or diffusion may be bound by charcoal and eliminated. Drug characteristics — low PB, small Vd, low Cl drugs, e.g. theophylline.

Drugs for which continuous oral charcoal may be useful
Theophylline
Phenobarbitone
Carbamazepine
Dioxins
Polychlorinated biphenyls

Haemodialysis: This may be useful in severe poisonings with dialysable drugs (low PB, small molecules) that have small Vd and meaningful enhancement in Cl, e.g. lithium.

Drugs for which haemodialysis is the method of choice in severe poisonings
Salicylates
Phenobarbitone
Lithium
Methanol
Ethanol
Ethylene glycol

Haemoperfusion: Blood is passed through adsorbent particles that bind and remove drug. May be more effective than haemodialysis and is not limited by high protein binding. Disadvantages include removal of blood contents, especially platelets and calcium.

Drugs for which haemoperfusion is the method of choice in severe poisoning
Theophylline
Barbiturates
Trichloroethanol derivatives

(iii) Antidotes

Specific antagonists are available for a few compounds. The effects may be dramatic.

NB: these are also potential toxins. Be aware of the time-course of action of these compared with the drug being treated, e.g. naloxone has a shorter $t_{1/2}$ than many narcotics and may need repeated dosing.

Drugs for which antidotes may be useful

Poison	Antidote
Cyanide	Dicobalt edetate
Carbon monoxide	Oxygen
Opiates	Naloxone
Benzodiazepine	Flumazenil
Paracetamol	N-acetyl cysteine
Iron	Desferriozamine
Organophosphate	Atropine
	Pralidoxime
Methanol	Ethanol
Ethylene glycol	Ethanol
Digoxin	Feb antibodies

4

Common Poisonings

	Major effects	Specific management
Aspirin (salicylates)	Acid–base disturbance Uncoupling oxidative phosphorylation Disordered glucose metabolism Resp. alkalosis/metabolic acidosis More dangerous in children	Measure serum salicylates Alkaline diuresis Haemodialysis
Benzodiazepines	CNS depression	Administer flumazenil (with repeats prn) for diagnosis and treatment
Carbon monoxide	Loss of functioning Hb Metabolic acidosis 'cherry pink' colour (carboxyhaemoglobin)	100% oxygen Hyperbaric oxygen
Cyanide	Inhibits cellular oxidation Metabolic acidosis 'Bitter almond' smell	Na thiosulphate: $CN \rightarrow SCN$ Amyl NO_2: metHb $\rightarrow$ CNmetHb Dicobalt edetate: chelation
Ethylene glycol	Inebriation Metabolic acidosis Hyperosmolality (osmolar gap) Pulmonary oedema	Measure serum concentrations Measure serum osmolality Ethanol infusion Haemodialysis
Lithium	GI symptoms CNS stimulation/coma Nephrotoxicity	Measure serum concentrations Haemodialysis
Methanol	Metabolic acidosis Hyperosmolality (osmolar gap)	Measure serum concentrations Measure serum osmolality Ethanol infusion Haemodialysis
Narcotics	Drowsiness or coma Pin-point pupils Respiratory depression	Naloxone IV — repeat often if necessary Monitoring ++
Organophosphates	Cholinergic effects Pulmonary oedema Convulsions	Atropine — antagonizes ACh Pralidoxine — reactivates acetylcholinesterases
Paracetamol	Symptoms often absent Hepatic necrosis Renal tubular necrosis	Measure serum concentrations N-acetylcysteine IV Monitoring ++

Continued

4

Continued

	Major effects	**Specific management**
Paraquat	Necrosis of lung (pulmonary fibrosis), kidney, liver, heart, adrenals	Measure serum concentrations Activated charcoal Fuller's earth Magnesium sulphate Oxygen contraindicated
Theophylline	GI symptoms Cardiac stimulation CNS stimulation Hypokalaemia	Activated charcoal Measure serum concentrations Supportive treatment Haemoperfusion
Tricyclics	Anticholinergic effects Metabolic acidosis CNS effects — excitability + coma Cardiotoxicity — ↑ HR, wide QRS	Activated charcoal Supportive treatment Serum concentrations sometimes helpful Monitor ICU

4

Pharmacological Aspects of Drug Dependence

> **Drug dependence**: 'Preoccupation with a drug to the detriment of other interests or responsibilities, and compulsion to take it without concern for the consequences.'

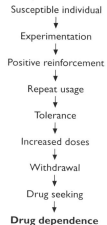

Drug dependence cascade

Susceptible individual
↓
Experimentation
↓
Positive reinforcement
↓
Repeat usage
↓
Tolerance
↓
Increased doses
↓
Withdrawal
↓
Drug seeking
↓
Drug dependence

Drugs involved

Psychoactive

- Opiates
- CNS stimulants
  amphetamines
  ecstacy (MDMA)
  cocaine
- Cannabis
- LSD
- Alcohol
- Nicotine
- CNS depressants
  benzodiazepines
  barbiturates
  GHB (gammahydroxybutyrate)
- Volatile substances — glue sniffing.

Sports enhancing (not discussed further)

- Anabolic steroids
- Erythropoietin
- Growth hormone
- Phenylpropanolamines
- β-Blockers.

Features of psychoactive drugs

(i) **Rapid delivery to brain:** The drugs are usually highly lipid soluble, well assimilated into the body and cross readily into the brain. Rapid assimilation is achieved by administration IV, or by inhalation.

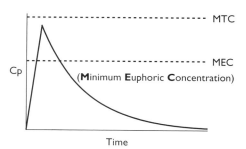

(ii) **Positive psychoactive effects:** The effects are reinforcing for that particular individual, e.g. euphoria, empowerment, disinhibition, heightened sensory awareness, calming effect (in stress).

(iii) **Tolerance:**
Constant dose → less effect
Larger dose → same effect
    Tolerance is greater with larger doses given for longer periods.
- **Metabolic tolerance** — Drug clearance increases through enzyme induction, caus-

ing lower concentrations for a given dose (i.e. autoinduction) i.e. same dose → less effect. Metabolic cross-tolerance can occur when induced enzymes metabolize other drugs.

• **Neuroadaptation** — With homeostasis, the body adapts to the 'insult', to return the settings to 'normal'. Adaptation occurs via receptor up- or down-regulation, alteration in membrane integrity, etc. The new setting requires drug to be present to maintain the newly acquired equilibrium. Increased doses are needed to achieve the reinforcing psychoactive effects. Cross-tolerance occurs between drugs with similar effects, e.g. alcohol/benzodiazepines.

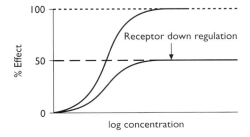

(iv) **Withdrawal symptoms**: 'the unopposed consequences of drug-induced neuroadaptation.' Absence of drug results in a 'deficiency state' characterized by symptoms opposite to those induced by the drug itself, e.g.

sedative withdrawal → agitation, seizures
stimulant withdrawal → sedation,
                                            depression

The *duration* of the withdrawal syndrome is directly related to the half-life of the drug and active metabolites, i.e.

longer $t_{1/2}$ → longer syndrome.

The *magnitude* of the withdrawal syndrome is inversely related to the $t_{1/2}$ of the drug, i.e.

shorter $t_{1/2}$ → more intense syndrome.

Pharmacological treatment of drug dependence

This is adjunctive to psychotherapy, behavioural modification, environmental modification, etc.

Many people have no trouble 'stopping', but more trouble 'quitting'.

(i) **Drug substitution therapy**: A similar drug with different pharmacokinetic properties (usually longer $t_{1/2}$) is used to decrease the intensity of, and to protract, the withdrawal process, e.g.

methadone for opiate addiction
benzodiazepines for alcohol withdrawal
nicotine patches for smoking

The dose of the substituted drug is then tapered in a controlled way.

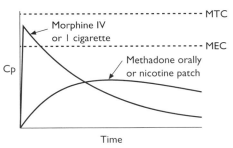

(ii) **Drug antagonist therapy**: After withdrawal has been completed, antagonists may prevent the reinforcing effects of a rechallenge, e.g. naltrexone versus heroin. There is little proof of the efficacy of this.

(iii) **Aversive therapy**: A drug may cause aversive symptoms if the drug of dependence is resumed, e.g. disulfiram/alcohol.

Perspective

From a global point of view, the damage caused by nicotine and alcohol far exceeds that of any other drug of abuse.

4

5 Optimal therapeutics

5

Principles of Drug Action

> Pharmacodynamics:
> 'What the drug does to the body'

The relationship between pharmacokinetics and pharmacodynamics is shown in the following diagram.

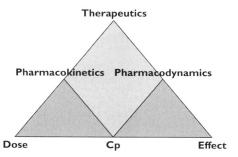

Concentration–Effect (C–E) relation

Drug effect cannot rise indefinitely as concentrations increase, e.g. an artery can only dilate to a certain extent or it will explode! It follows that the relationship between concentration and effect cannot be linear, but follows a curve as shown.

NB: C, rather than Cp, is used for the concentrations since this is the concentration at the site of activity (the **biophase**).

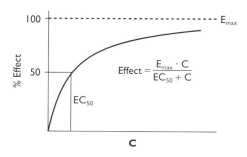

$$Effect = \frac{E_{max} \cdot C}{EC_{50} + C}$$

This curve is analogous, and functionally related, to receptor occupancy. As receptor occupancy by drug approaches total occupancy, maximum **effect** (E_{max}) is reached. The concentration at which 50% effect

occurs is called EC_{50} (effective concentration, 50%) and is an index of **potency**. These terms may be understood more easily with graphs using the log of the concentration.

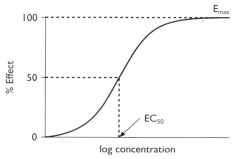

Effect (or efficacy) and potency are different concepts. Maximum effect defines the ultimate achievable response, while potency defines the dose at which responses occur. A full agonist has greater efficacy than a partial agonist independent of potency, e.g. morphine (full opiate agonist) is a better analgesic than buprenorphine (partial agonist). However, buprenorphine (usual oral dose 0.2 mg) is more potent than morphine (usual oral dose 10 mg).

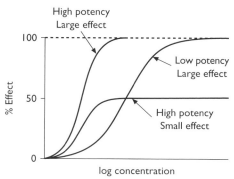

From the shape of the concentration–effect curve, it can be seen that the 'law of diminishing returns' applies.

Law of diminishing returns

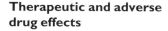

C	Effect (%)	Gain (%)
$1 \times EC_{50}$	50	50
$2 \times EC_{50}$	67	17
$3 \times EC_{50}$	75	8
$4 \times EC_{50}$	80	5
$9 \times EC_{50}$	90	10

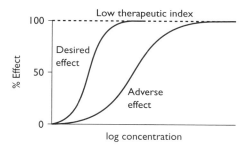

Therapeutic and adverse drug effects

There are separate concentration–effect curves for desired (therapeutic) and undesired (adverse) effects. Hopefully for most drugs the EC_{50} for desired effects is considerably lower than that of undesired effects, i.e. there is a large **therapeutic index**.

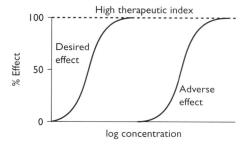

If this is so, dosing is easy. However, many drugs have a low therapeutic index (e.g. cancer chemotherapy) and there is a thin line between the good and the bad.

The site of the 'effect compartment'

Some drugs act in the 'central' compartment. Their effects will therefore relate directly to the plasma concentration. If, however, the biophase is somewhere out in the tissues, then the concentration in that peripheral compartment is relevant, and not the Cp.

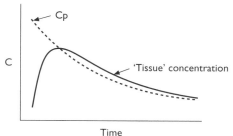

Dose and dose interval should be titrated to achieve desired concentrations in the effect compartment.

Applied Pharmacology

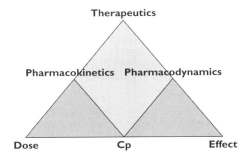

Pharmacodynamic considerations

Concentration–effect curves look simple, but normal variation suggests that the E_{max} and the EC_{50} will vary considerably between individuals. This needs to be taken into account in dosing.

Some people will get a good response at a very low concentration, while others will require a higher concentration. Some people, even after dose escalation, never achieve an adequate response, and may require a different type of drug.

The approach to dosing depends on the therapeutic situation, the therapeutic index of the drug and on the shape of the dose–response curve. If the drug has a high therapeutic index, e.g. penicillin, then it is reasonable to give a big dose early on so that the chances of success are very high, e.g. a dose designed to be sure of maximum effect in everyone. If the drug has a low therapeutic index, e.g. digoxin, it is important to dose more cautiously and titrate to desired response.

The more urgent a situation, the more 'risk' can be tolerated, e.g. it may be necessary to load digoxin to control a tachyarrhythmia even though some patients might experience some nausea.

Tachyphylaxis/tolerance

Response may change with time, usually as a homeostatic response of the body to the 'intrusion' of the drug.

Tachyphylaxis (= 'quick protection') refers to a rapid diminution in response to a drug, usually within minutes or hours. Response also returns rapidly on removal of the drug, e.g. nitrates in angina. The mechanism is usually depletion of a secondary messenger, or receptor internalization, (i.e. the receptors are temporarily 'removed' from exposure to the drug by reorientation to face inside the cell membrane rather than outside).

Tolerance refers to a more gradual decline in effectiveness of a drug, usually over days or weeks. It is reflected in increasing dose requirements, e.g. opiates in drug addiction. The mechanism is usually a change in receptor number (up or down-regulation), or the development of an opposing physiological response, e.g. Na^+ and water retention with a vasodilator. The time-course of reversal is similar to that of onset.

'Withdrawal/rebound'

Withdrawal symptoms are the unopposed consequences of drug-induced physiological adaptation. The absence of the drug results in a 'deficiency state' characterized by symptoms opposite to those induced by the drug itself, e.g. after withdrawal of β-blockers, rebound hypertension or angina/myocardial infarction can occur, as a result of unmasking of up-regulated β-receptor numbers. Ceasing drugs can be very dangerous and should be undertaken slowly and judiciously.

Pharmacokinetic considerations

Loading doses

Vd determines the size of the loading dose. The Vd is often disturbed in sick people because of dysfunction of biological barriers, e.g. larger Vd of antibiotics in infection.

Maintenance doses

Cl, the determinant of the maintenance dose, may be altered by age, disease states, other drugs, genetics or autoinduction/autoinhibition. Variation *between* individuals needs to be considered at the time the maintenance dose is initiated, while variation *within* individuals is important thereafter.

Dose interval

The $t_{1/2}$ is the major pharmacokinetic determinant of the dose interval, although many other factors, such as compliance, therapeutic index of the drug, the locus of the effect compartment, and the mode of administration (e.g. tablet, slow-release preparation, IV infusion, etc.) are also important. A drug with a $t_{1/2}$ that allows once or twice daily dosing is good for compliance.

Therapeutic plan

The therapeutic plan embraces all of the above, but also takes into account therapeutic objectives, monitoring and possible dose tapering. The therapeutic plan needs to be revised any time the condition changes or a new drug is added or deleted.

Dose tapering

Upon achievement of the therapeutic objective (e.g. attainment of a target BP), it may be possible to back-titrate the dose until control deteriorates again, then increasing the dose slightly. In this way the minimum dose that achieves the desired effect can be approached.

> The concept of a single dose for everyone is pharmacologically naive. **Treat the individual**

Compliance with Medication

Compliance and non-compliance mean 'success or failure in following instructions'

Non-compliance is probably the biggest problem in therapeutics. Very few people take a full course of medication exactly as prescribed, e.g. how many of us actually complete a course of antibiotics exactly as prescribed? Failure to achieve the desired therapeutic endpoint as a result of non-compliance occurs in 30–50% of treatment courses.

One problem with compliance is the term itself. It is too authoritarian. An alternative term, 'adherence', has been used as a substitute, but is little better. Recently 'concordance' has been proposed as a better term as it embraces an agreement between the patient and the doctor, about the proposed plan.

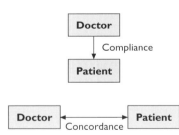

Reasons for non-compliance

- Patients do not want to be sick
- Patients may not want to take drugs
- Patients may fear the (perhaps unknown) effects of long-term therapy
- Cost
- Inconvenience
- Complexity.

A less patronizing approach by doctors, recognizing that non-compliance should actually be expected, is likely to reap dividends.

Promoting compliance

(i) The patient (the central figure)

It is important to recognize the patient's need for self-determination. An appropriate educational strategy for each patient needs to be devised, taking into account their level of understanding and potential barriers to compliance. Compliance aids should be provided if appropriate.

(ii) The prescription (things you should think about)

- Is the drug really necessary?
- Use as few drugs as possible, for as short a time as possible.
- Regularly review drug therapy.
- Do not change long-term therapy without good cause.
- Use once-daily or twice-daily dosing regimens where possible.
- Provide medication chart if >2 drugs, or in elderly / confused patients.
- If titrating, provide specific instructions (e.g. asthma plan).
- Use consistent names (e.g. generic).

(iii) Medication details (give to patient verbally, and as patient information leaflets [PILs])

- Name of medication and why given.
- How and when to take it.
- What to do if dose missed.
- How long to take it.
- Benefits expected and when they will occur.
- Possible problems to expect (e.g. side effects).

- How to manage side-effects.
- Food/drinks/other drugs (including over the counter) to avoid.
- How to obtain further information.
- Follow-up appointment for review.

Education/compliance aids
(see Patients and their drugs, page 80)

- Patient Information Leaflets (PILs).
- Medication charts ('Yellow cards').
- Pill organizers.

Detecting non-compliance

- Expect it!
- Discuss it openly.
- Assess extent (e.g. total non-compliance vs occasional missed doses).
- Avoid imposing guilt — generalize the problem and offer excuses for the patient.
- Take blame yourself.

Managing non-compliance

- Discuss the good and not so good about taking medication.
- Negotiate (as part of the concordance strategy) e.g. 'Where do you want to go from here?'.
- Make a realistic contract (the agreement) with realistic goals, e.g. 'Do the best as you see it.'
- Review — establish specific time, place and person.
- Elicit help — nurse and pharmacist.

1   Recognize that compliance is a problem
2   Redefine it as 'concordance'
3   Make an effort to address it

5

Principles of Therapeutics

1 Accurate diagnosis
• Without an accurate diagnosis all therapeutic endeavours are inappropriate.

2 Is drug therapy necessary?
• Remediable causes of disease should be addressed first, e.g. smoking, alcohol, obesity, high-fat diet.

3 Choose the right drug
• What is the best theoretical drug for the condition?
• How good is the evidence?
• Is this drug appropriate for this patient?
(Examine the patient profile and the drug profile).

4 Use the drug correctly
• Is a loading dose necessary?
• Should the starting dose be low?
• What is the usual maintenance dose?
• Is this dose appropriate for this patient?
  adjust for age?
  adjust for renal dysfunction?
  adjust for liver dysfunction?
  adjust for drug interactions?
• What is the best dose interval?
• Which route of administration?

5 Define therapeutic objectives
• Cure? e.g. antibiotic for infection
• Relieve symptoms? e.g. palliative care for cancer
• Replace deficiencies? e.g. insulin for diabetes.

6 Monitor drug effect
• Measure desired end-point (e.g. BP)
• Side effects
• Measure drug concentrations.

7 Duration of therapy
• Single dose? e.g. sumatriptan
• Short course? e.g. antibiotics
• For life? e.g. antihypertensives.

8 Promote compliance
• Talk to patient about their drugs
• Keep drug regimen simple
• Compliance aids
• 'Concordance'.

9 Know your drugs
• Use a few drugs well rather than many badly.

10 Therapeutic parsimony
• Use the lowest dose of as few drugs for as short as possible to achieve the desired effect.

11 Review therapy
• at time of new consultations
• on admission to hospital
• whenever adding new drugs
• when anything untoward occurs.

12 Avoid overprescribing
• antibiotics for viral infections
• antidepressants for normal life situations
• sedatives for occasional sleep disturbance
• vitamins when diet adequate.

13 Avoid underprescribing
• narcotics (fear of addiction)
• antidepressants (fear of disease label)
• aminoglycosides (underdosage for fear of toxicity).

14 Accurate prescription
• Clear
• Concise
• Correct
• Complete.

Essentials of a good prescription

A prescription is a written communication. It is vitally important that the information transmitted within a prescription is accur-ate, unambiguous, and complete. Where ambiguity is possible, write details in full. The prescriber's name must be recognizable, and he/she readily traceable.

Physician's name and registration number	Dr A Prescriber LN2693
Address	10 Dispensary Drive Drugsville
Phone number	(03) 271 8281
Patient Name	Mrs May B Compliant
Address	39 Tempup Lane Illsbury
Date of birth (preferable)	9/5/45
Date:	01/01/01
Rx: Drug name (preferably generic, and UPPER CASE), dose and strength	AMOXYCILLIN, 250 mg tablets
Directions for administration	Take one t.d.s. p.o. with food
Quantity to be dispensed	15
Any specific instructions	Take until course finished
Any repeats	Nil
Prescriber's signature:	*A Prescriber*
Prescriber's name in UPPER CASE	A PRESCRIBER

5

Patients and their Drugs

Patient outcomes and compliance can be improved greatly if attention is paid to all aspects of communication between them and their health professional about their drugs.

Taking a drug history — What to ask patients about their drugs.
1 What drugs are you currently taking?
2 How long have you been taking them?
3 What doses, and how frequently?
4 Have there been benefits from them?
5 Any side effects?
6 What drugs have you had previously for the same condition(s)?
7 Why did you stop these?
8 Are you taking any other drugs?
   regularly?
   occasionally?
   forgotten 'drugs' e.g. oral contraceptives?
   purchased over the counter?
   herbal or alternative medicines?
9 Do you have any drug allergies/intolerances?
10 Alcohol/smoking/illegal drug history.

Patient education — What to tell the patient about their drugs.
1 Name of the medication
2 Why it has been prescribed
3 How and when to take it
4 How long it should be taken for
5 Benefits expected and when they might occur
6 Possible problems to expect, and how to deal with them
7 Food/drink/other drugs (including over the counter) to avoid
8 What to do if a dose is missed
9 How to obtain further information
10 Follow-up appointment for review.

Discharge prescribing — How to make things easier for the patient.

Information/devices that should be given to appropriate patients at the time of discharge or at the end of an out-patient appointment.
1 Changes made to the medication regimen
2 Any dose changes required (e.g. reducing doses of corticosteroids)
3 An unambiguous prescription (helps pharmacist, and indirectly the patient)
   Clear
   Concise
   Complete
   Written in Capitals
   Prescriber identifiable
4 A medication card
5 A unit dose packaging device
6 Patient information leaflets.

Medication card

A medication card (locally called the 'yellow card') is a useful reminder to the patient of what drugs they are taking, when and why. They are good for any patient with complex or multiple prescriptions, especially the aged and the infirm. They should be carried by the patient whenever possible, and certainly to any visits to medical, paramedical personnel or hospital.

Medications cards may contain the following information:
• Name of patient
• Any allergies
• Name of patient's regular (primary) doctor
• Drug name
• Drug form and strength
• Dosage and time taken (e.g. breakfast, dinner, lunch)
• Purpose of drug
• Special instructions.

Unit dose packaging devices

Drug administration devices in which drugs are organized into convenient compartments are useful to assist ordered drug compliance, e.g. drugs taken at breakfast time will be in one compartment. These are particularly useful for patients with multiple medications, those who might forget to take their medications, and those (e.g. patients with arthritis) who cannot open pill bottles.

Patient information leaflets (PILs)

There is increasing pressure, both medically and legally, for patients to be given simple, written information about their drugs that they can take away and refer to in their own time. This is because it is impossible for patients to remember all the information given to them at the time of discharge or at the end of a consultation. The information should be written as simply as possible, usually aiming for a reading age of about 10 years. PILs that have been prepared by pharmacy/clinical staff with great attention to presentation style and simplicity are the best.

Information contained in PILs may include:
• Drug name (generic and trade)
• What does it do?
• How it should be taken (e.g. with food, with water etc.)
• What to do if a dose is forgotten
• Can other medicines be taken (including herbal and OTC)
• Side effects and recommended action if they occur
• Other information.

5

The Drug Profile

Each drug has its own **drug profile**, all aspects of which are considered in relation to the **patient profile** during prescribing.

The drug profile is made up of the following major headings.

> Drug name (generic)
> Class/therapeutic category
> Action
> Pharmacokinetics
> Factors affecting pharmacokinetics
> Indications (registered/unregistered)
> Contraindications/precautions
> Adverse reactions
> Interactions
> Dosing information
> Monitoring
> Overdose (symptoms/signs/treatment)

A consistent template approach to formulating drug profiles assists in both transmission of drug information and the learning process.

Most modern information sources follow a fairly uniform template pattern in their approach to providing drug information (see Drug Information/Resources, page 88).

An example of a drug profile is printed on the facing page.

<u>FLUOXETINE</u>
(Prozac™, Lovan™)

Class:	Selective Serotonin Reuptake Inhibitor (SSRI)
Action:	*Major*: antidepressant
	Minor: inhibits reuptake of 5-HT at synapses

Pharmacokinetics: Oral availability: >0.6 (first-pass)   Vd: 2450 L/70 kg (770–3290)

P.B: 0.94 $t_{1/2}$: 53 hr (12–94) [6.4±2.5days — norfluoxetine]

fu: < 0.03   Cl: 40 L/hr/70 kg (11–69)

Metabolism: CYP2D6, 3A4

FLUOXETINE → NORFLUOXETINE → INACTIVE METABOLITES
            CYP2D6   (active)   CYP3A4

Factors affecting   Hepatic disease: ↓ Cl in cirrhosis
pharmacokinetics: Genetics: subject to CYP2D6 polymorphism
                                              (5–10% Caucasian, 1–3% Asians slow)

Indications: depression*, obsessive compulsive disorder*, bulimia*, ?panic disorder,
(* registered)   premenstrual tension

Contraindications/   MAOIs, ↓ dose in liver disease
Precautions: *Pregnancy*:   FDA — B [Animal studies haven't shown a risk but no controlled
                                        studies in humans OR animal studies have shown an ADR not
                                        confirmed in controlled studies in women in 1st trim + no evidence
                                        of risk in later trimesters'; 1st trim — ↑ spontaneous abortions; 3rd trim
                                        — perinatal complications]
                           Lactation: % maternal dose (wt adjusted): 6–13% [includes norfluoxetine and
                                        fluoxetine]

Adverse reactions: >10%   CNS: headache, nervousness, insomnia, drowsiness
                                   GI: nausea, diarrhoea, dry mouth
                           1–10%   CNS: anxiety, dizziness, fatigue, sedation
                                   Endo: SIADH, hypoglycaemia, hyponatraemia
                                   GI: anorexia, dyspepsia, constipation
                                   Misc: sweating, rash, pruritis, tremor, sexual dysfunction, weight loss
                           <1%   Misc: extrapyramidal reactions, anaphylactoid reactions, allergies, visual
                                        disturbances, suicidal ideation

Interactions: Many interactions:
                           Pharmacokinetic:
                           CYP2D6 inhibition: ↑ Cp of diazepam, lipophilic β-blockers, antipsychotics
                           CYP2C9 inhibition: ↑ warfarin Cp. *NB*. Also antiplatelet effect — ↑ bleeding
                           Also inhibits CYP3A3/4 therefore ↑ Cp terfenadine, cisapride etc.
                           Pharmacodynamic:
                           Serotonin syndrome with other 5-HT enhancers (e.g. MAOIs, TCAs, Lithium, 5-HT
                           precursors, St John's wort)

Dosing: 20–80 mg/day. Higher for bulimia?
Monitoring: Adverse reactions, serum Na$^+$
Overdose: *Signs/symptoms*: potentially dangerous in overdose — serotonin syndrome
                           particularly in combination with other 5-HT enhancers (see list above in
                           interactions).
                           Treatment: supportive

5

Evidence-based Medicine

> The explicit and judicious use of current best evidence in making decisions about the care of individual patients.
>
> Sackett *et al.*, *Evidence-Based Medicine*. New York, NY: Churchill Livingstone; 1997.

There is an increasing expectation for healthcare professionals to practise 'evidence-based medicine'. At the same time, the increasing volume and complexity of information, in the setting of time constraints, makes this very difficult. Further, as in criminal law, there are various degrees of evidence. 'Truth' is hard to find.

Evidence-based medicine is a laudable concept with natural appeal, that has itself become quite an industry (e.g. Cochrane collaboration). Used correctly, it is an essential guide to patient management. Misused, it can approach a religion, and mislead.

It is important to maintain a healthy scepticism not only about the evidence itself, but also about the doctrine of evidence-based medicine.

Evaluation of scientific evidence
1 Identify the specific clinical concern
2 Retrieve all contributory information
3 Categorize studies according to their strength of evidence
4 Use all of the 'best' studies to derive clinical recommendations.

Strength of evidence (decreasing order)
I Randomized controlled trials (RCTs)
II Controlled trials without randomization
III Cohort, case-control or cross-sectional studies
IV Uncontrolled studies
V Descriptive studies/opinion.

In reality, scientific support for a notion is often conflicting or absent. The evidence-based approach should recognize this and make use of all the information that is available. If there is no robust RCT available to answer a question (very common), this is not an excuse to ignore all the information that does exist.

The Randomized Controlled Trial (RCT): This remains the Gold Standard, even if it is far from perfect.
Key features:
• Uniform patient selection — strict inclusion and exclusion criteria ensure maximum chance of detecting 'signal' from 'noise'.
• Randomization — to active (new drug) or control (placebo or active comparator) groups.
• Blinding — usually 'double-blind', which means both patient and observer do not know which patient is in which group.
Problems:
• Lack of generalizability — patient selection is stringent and therefore the results may not apply to your patient.
• Artificial clinical environment — the patients is treated by a highly motivated researcher who does not know which compound the patient is receiving, and has little flexibility in dosage adjustment etc.
• Blinding is rarely possible — drugs have effects that are discerned by both patient and observer, e.g. slowed pulse with β-blocker.

Meta-analysis: This is a complicated statistical technique for pooling the data from multiple similar clinical trials, in order to increase the statistical power. It has its own problems including generalizing results from trials with different methodologies, subjective selection of trials to be included, and 'publication bias' (negative trials are less likely to be published, increasing the likelihood of a positive net outcome).

Controlled trials without randomization: These are similar to RCTs, but patients are not truly randomized, e.g. every alternate patient may enter respective groups. These are weaker than RCTs.

Cohort studies: These track people *forward* in time, from exposure to outcome. Exposed and unexposed groups are followed to see if outcomes differ. They are slow and expensive.

Case–control studies: These track people *backwards* from outcome to exposure. Groups with and without a condition are examined retrospectively to see if proposed risk factors differed in prevalence. While more efficient than cohort studies, it is difficult to choose a truly equivalent control group.

Cross-sectional studies: These are a snap-shot (prevalence study) of outcome and exposure at a single time-point. They are easy to conduct.

Descriptive studies: These merely describe the characteristics of a condition. They may lead to hypotheses that can be tested more formally to establish causal association.

Statistical analysis: Confidence intervals (often but not necessarily the 95% limits) around measures distinguishing index and control groups indicates the precision and chance of the results. They are preferred over p-values, which address only chance at an arbitrary value.

'Let us agree that good clinical medicine will always blend the art of uncertainty with the science of probability. But let us also hope that the blend can be weighted heavily towards science, whenever and wherever evidence is brought to light.'

William Osler

5

Pharmacoeconomics

> Pharmacoeconomics is about maximizing the net benefits of the drugs purchased by society

Health resources are never unlimited. Allocation decisions must be made, and pharmacoeconomics provides a framework for this. It is **not** a system for reducing costs.

The science of pharmacoeconomics is imperfect, and uncertainty abounds. This is reflected by the different perspectives, biases and abilities of the analysts, the various types of analyses used, and the subjectivity involved in many of the assessments. This very looseness allows for potential misuse of the components of the process, and abuse of the outcomes.

Perspectives

Pharmacoeconomic analysis can be undertaken from a variety of perspectives.
- Society
- Patient
- Provider
- Drug company.

The widest perspective, and therefore usually the best, is that of society as a whole. It is easy to see the potential biases of the other perspectives.

Types of pharmacoeconomic analysis

Cost-minimization analysis (CMA): This approach may be used when alternative therapies have identical outcomes (well established) but differ in costs. The measure is simply cost. The best treatment is the cheapest.

Cost-effectiveness analysis (CEA): This may be used when alternative therapies dif-fer in their clinical effectiveness on a single health outcome, and also differ in costs. Superior efficacy is weighed against increased costs. The measure is the C/E ratio (cost to effectiveness), e.g. cost per life saved.

Cost–utility analysis (CUA): This is similar to CEA but the alternative therapies are compared against multiple outcomes (e.g. effectiveness, morbidity, mortality). Each outcome may be weighted by patient preference. The summarized measure of effectiveness is the QALY (quality adjusted life years). The measure is the C/E ratio, where E is the QALY.

Cost–benefit analysis (CBA): This compares benefits, expressed in monetary terms, with costs. The measure is the B/C ratio (benefits to costs).

Which is best?

The CUA is the most universal, and therefore overall the best approach. However, it requires more information, more assumptions and more subjectivity, so unless the data is good the results may mislead, i.e. garbage in, garbage out!

What are costs?

Costs may be direct, indirect, or intangible.
- *Direct costs*: These include the actual cost of the drugs and everything associated with their delivery. E.g. diagnostic tests, monitoring, treating side effects.
- *Indirect costs*: These include days lost from work/school, or lost employment opportunities, e.g. through arthritis.
- *Intangible costs*: These include less definable things such as pain and suffering.

It is clear that many of these costs are very difficult to quantify accurately.

How is the pharmacoeconomic analysis performed?

There are various models, mostly computer based, including decision trees, Markov diagrams and other complex algorithms that I do not understand! These are specialized tools that require expert knowledge.

How to manage uncertainty

This is done by a technique called 'sensitivity analysis'. Values of the various parameters in the model are altered to see how this affects the overall decision. In this way unimportant parameters can be identified and ignored.

Unless the evidence basis, assumptions, biases and uncertainties are stated very explicitly, the results of pharmacoeconomic studies should be treated with great caution

Checklist for evaluating pharmacoeconomic studies

1 Are the aims clearly stated?
2 Are the alternative therapies clearly defined?
3 Is the perspective of the analyst apparent, and appropriate?
4 Is the type of analysis appropriate?
5 Have all outcomes been identified and measured?
6 Have all costs been identified and measured?
7 Has sensitivity analysis been performed?
8 Have all assumptions been defined explicitly?
9 Are the results presented clearly and fairly?
10 Are the conclusions justified?

5

Drug Information/ Resources

The basis of good prescribing is the ready availability of good drug information

The ideal is to have comprehensive information available at 'time of need'. This is usually at the time of writing a prescription.

Information available to health professionals can be thought of in three tiers:

1 Instantly available (portable, on desk): These include local guidelines, preferred medicines lists, national formularies, drug information handbooks, and computerized databases (including palmtop). These contain 'drug profile' information for routine prescribing, such as:

• Mechanism of action
• Pharmacokinetics
• Factors altering pharmacokinetics
• Indications
• Contraindications/precautions
• Adverse drug effects
• Interactions
• Dosing information
• Monitoring
• Overdose.

Some useful resources include:
• British National Formulary
• Australian Medicines Handbook
• Drug Information Handbook
• Epocrates
• Drdrugs.

2 Readily available (in wards, in group practice libraries, in dispensaries): These include larger resources with more detailed information about the same general areas of the drug profile. They include large comput-

erized databases that provide access to the major world literature, to provide 'evidence-based medicine'.

Some useful resources include:
• Martindale — The Complete Drug Reference
• American Hospital Formulary Service (AHFS)
• Drug Interactions, Stockley
• Drugdex System, Micromedex 2002
• Medline CD ROM
• Embase CD ROM.

3 At libraries/drug information services: These include specialist texts covering highly specific details in relevant areas of interest (e.g. drugs in pregnancy or lactation, drug interactions, adverse drug reactions).

Some useful resources include:
• *Therapeutic Drugs*, Dollery
• *Goodman and Gilman's The Pharmacological Basis of Therapeutics*
• *Avery's Drug Treatment*
• *Davies's Textbook of Adverse Drug Reactions*
• *Meyler's Side Effects of Drugs*
• *Drugs and Human Lactation*, Bennett
• *Drugs in Pregnancy and Lactation*, Briggs.

Types of questions asked of a drug information service

Analysis of our own drug information service database reveals that the majority of questions come from the following categories. This may indicate where resources should be directed.

Category	% total
Adverse reactions	21
Contraindications/precautions	20
Drug interactions	19
Administration/dosage	13
Drug choice/selection	7
Other	20

Useful further information on pharmacology/clinical pharmacology

Clinical Pharmacokinetics, Rowland, M. and Tozer, N. 3rd ed. (1995). Williams & Wilkins, London.

Pharmacokinetics made easy, Birkett, D.J. (1999). McGraw Hill, Sydney

Pharmacology, Raffa, R.B. (1999). Blackwell Science, Oxford.

How to access the resources

British National Formulary (2001). British Medical Association and Royal Pharmaceutical Association of Great Britain.

Australian Medicines Handbook 2nd ed. (2002). Australian Medical Handbook Pty Ltd, P.O. Box 240, Rundle Mall, Adelaide, South Australia.

Drug Information Handbook, Lacy, C.F., Armstrong, L.L., Goldman, M.P. and Lance, L.L. 9th ed. (2001–2002). Lexicomp Inc., Hudson, Cleveland.

Epocrates (Palm OS) www.epocrates.com

Drdrugs (Win CE) www.skyscape.com

Martindale — The Complete Drug Reference 33rd ed. (2002). Pharmaceutical Press, London.

American Hospital Formulary Service (AHFS) (2002). AHFS, Washington.

Drug Interactions, Stockley, I.H. 5th ed. (1999). Pharmaceutical Press, London.

Drugdex System, Micromedex 2002 Healthcare Series, Computer program.

Medline CD-ROM, 1966–2002.

Embase CD-ROM, 1988–2002.

Therapeutic Drugs, Dollery, C. 2nd ed. (1999). Churchill Livingstone, Edinburgh.

Goodman and Gilman's — The Pharmacological Basis of Therapeutics, 10th ed. (2002) (ed. Hardman *et al.*) McGraw Hill, New York.

Avery's Drug Treatment 4th ed. (1997). Adis International, Auckland.

Davies's Textbook of Adverse Drug Reactions 5th ed. (1998). Chapman & Hall, London.

Meyler's Side Effects of Drugs 14th ed. (2000). Elsevier, Amsterdam.

Drugs and Human Lactation, Bennett, P.N. 2nd ed. (1996). Elsevier, Oxford.

Drugs in Pregnancy and Lactation, Briggs, G.G. 5th ed. (1998). Williams & Wilkins, Baltimore.

5

6 Appendix

6

Important Equations in Pharmacology

Vd

$$Ab = Vd * Cp \text{ or } Vd = \frac{Ab}{Cp}$$

F

$$F = \frac{AUC_{po}}{AUC_{iv}}$$

$$\text{Loading dose} = Vd * Cp_{desired}$$

CrCl

$$CrCl \text{ (mL/s)} = \frac{(140-age) * weight[kg]}{50\,000 * [creatinine]}$$
$$(* 0.85 \text{ for women})$$

Cl

$$RE = Cl * Cp \text{ or } Cl = \frac{RE}{Cp}$$

Dose adjustment in renal failure

$$\text{Maintenance dose} = Cl * Cp$$

$$\frac{dose \ rate_{patient}}{*dose \ rate_{normal}} = \frac{CrCl_{patient}}{CrCl_{normal}}$$

$$Cl = \frac{F * Dose}{AUC}$$

Dose adjustment in renal failure when fu < 1

$t_{1/2}$

$$t_{1/2} = \frac{0.693Vd}{Cl}$$

$$\frac{dose \ rate_{patient}}{*dose \ rate_{normal}} = (1 - fu) + fu \times \left(\frac{CrCl_{patient}}{CrCl_{normal}} \right)$$

6

The Pharmacokinetic Triangle

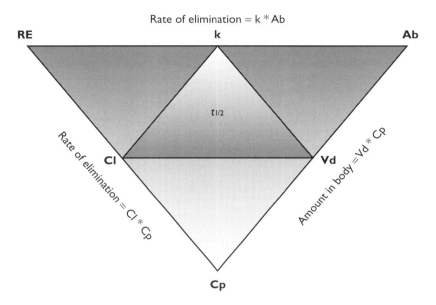

Glossary/Abbreviations

Ab: Amount of drug in the body.

ADE: Adverse drug event. Any actual or potential damage resulting from medical intervention related to medicines.

ADR: Adverse drug reaction. Any response to a drug which is noxious, unintended, and occurs at doses used in man for prophylaxis, diagnosis or therapy.

AUC: Area under the plasma, usually plasma curve concentration vs time curve.

Biophase: The immediate vicinity of the site of activity of a drug.

CBA: Cost-benefit analysis.

CEA: Cost-effectiveness analysis.

Clearance: The volume of plasma cleared of drug per unit time.
Or,
A constant relating the rate of elimination to the plasma concentration.

Clinical pharmacology: The principles behind the prescribing process.

CMA: Cost-minimization analysis.

C_{max}: Maximum concentration.

Compliance: In drug therapy this describes how much a patient is able to follow a full course of medication exactly as prescribed.

Concordance: This is the more modern, less authoritarian, interpretation of compliance that recognizes that a prescription embraces an agreement between the patient and the doctor.

Cp: Plasma concentration.

Cp_o: Plasma concentration at time zero.

Cp_{ss}: Plasma concentration at steady state.

Cp_t: Plasma concentration at time t.

CrCl: Creatinine clearance.

CUA: Cost-utility analysis.

CYP: Cytochrome P450.

Dose interval: The time interval between administration of doses.

Dose tapering: Back-titration of a dose of a drug after effect has been achieved, in order to achieve the minimum dose commensurate with desired effect.

e: The natural logarithm (value = 2.7183).

EC_{50}: The concentration of a drug at which effect is 50% maximum.

E_{max}: The maximum effect of a drug.

F: fractional oral availability.

First-order: A number to the power of one. In pharmacokinetics, it refers to elimination that is dependent on concentration (i.e. $Cp^1 = Cp$), as occurs with most drugs.

First-pass metabolism: Metabolism that occurs between the gut and the systemic circulation during the first passage of the drug through the portal system and the liver to the inferior vena cava.

Flow-dependent elimination: The elimination of high clearance drugs is so rapid that it is susceptible to the rate of presentation to the eliminating organ, and hence to blood flow.

fu: fraction excreted unchanged by the kidney.

Half-life: The time for the concentration of the drug in the plasma (or the amount of drug in the body) to halve.

k: rate constant of elimination: the fraction of drug removed per unit time. Applies to drugs with first-order elimination (i.e. most drugs).

Km: The Michealis constant. The concentration at which the rate of reaction is half the Vmax.

ln: the natural logarithm.

Loading dose: The dose required to achieve a target plasma concentration as soon as possible.

M/P ratio: Milk to plasma ratio.

MEC: Minimal effective concentration.

MTC: Minimal toxic concentration.

OTC: Over the counter.

P.B.: Protein Binding — usually expressed as a fraction or percentage.

pH: The negative of the log (base 10) of the concentration of hydrogen ions.

Pharmacodynamics: The study of drug effect, and mechanisms of action, i.e. What the drug does to the body.

Pharmacokinetics: The study of the movement of drugs into, within, and out of the body. i.e. what the body does to the drug.

Phase I metabolism: Simple chemical alteration of a molecule by oxidation (most commonly), reduction or hydrolysis. It occurs often by cytochrome p450 enzymes.

Phase II metabolism: Conjugation reactions including glucuronidation (most commonly), acetylation, sulphation and methylation.

pH-dependent elimination: Varying renal elimination of drugs with susceptible pKa values whose degree of ionization varies within the range of pH values of the urine (pH 4.5–8).

PILs: Patient information leaflets.

pKa: The pH at which a drug is 50% ionized, and 50% unionized.

Potency: An index of the concentration of a drug required for a given effect. The lower the concentration the greater the potency.

Prodrug: A drug that is inactive in itself, but which is converted to an active metabolite.

QALY: Quality adjusted life years.

RCT: Randomized controlled trial.

Saturable metabolism: Drug concentrations rise disproportionately as a result of a change from first-order to zero-order elimination.

SIADH: Syndrome of inappropriate antidiuretic hormone.

ss: Steady state

$T_{1/2}$: The half life.

Tachyphylaxis: Literally means 'quick protection'. It refers to a rapid diminution of response to a drug, usually within minutes or hours.

TDM: Therapeutic drug monitoring. Refers to the monitoring of drug concentrations as a surrogate for true pharmacodynamic end-points.

Teratogenicity: Literally means propensity to form a 'monster'. It refers to the propensity of a drug to cause a fetal malformation.

Therapeutic index: The ratio of concentration associated with toxicity vs efficiency.

Therapeutic range: The range of drug concentrations associated with a reasonable probability of efficacy, without undue toxicity in the majority of patients.

Therapeutics: The process of medical treatment.

T_{max}: Time to maximum concentration.

Tolerance: A gradual decline in effectiveness of a drug, usually over days or weeks, as a result of compensatory homeostasis (often receptor up or down regulation).

V_{max}: The maximum velocity of a chemical reaction.

Volume of distribution: The volume into which a drug appears to distribute with a concentration equal to that of plasma.
Or,
A proportionality constant relating the plasma concentration to the amount of drug in the body.

Zero-order: A number to the power of zero (i.e. always equals one i.e. $X^0 = 1$). In pharmacokinetics, it refers to elimination independent of concentration (i.e. $Cp^0 = 1$), as occurs with ethanol.

6

Test Questions

Answers are on page 98.

1 Pharmacokinetics

Cephazolin, 1000 mg, is given intravenously to a patient at 12:00 h as a 5-minute 'push'. The following concentration-time data was collected.

Time (h)	Concentration (mg/L)
12:30	76
13:00	58
14:00	46
16:00	22
18:00	12

(i)   Plot the data on semi-log paper.
(ii) Calculate the patient's Vd.
(iii) Calculate the $t_{1/2}$.
(iv) Calculate the AUC.
(v)   Calculate the Cl.

2 Loading and maintenance doses

You prescribe theophylline to a 28-year-old, 50 kg asthmatic. The target concentration is 15 mg/L.
(i) Calculate the loading dose.
(ii) Calculate the maintenance dose.

Assume:

• Vd = 0.5 L/kg
• Cl = 0.04 (L/h)/kg.

3 Dosing in altered metabolism

The metabolism of theophylline is induced by around 100% in smokers. The average maintenance dose to achieve a Cp of 10 mg/L in a non-smoker is 500 mg theophylline per day.

What maintenance dose would be needed in a smoker to achieve a Cp of 15 mg/L?

4 Saturable kinetics

A 5th-year medical student (70 kg) drinks eight 100 mL glasses of wine in one hour (naughty, naughty!). How long after starting to drink does he have to wait before it is 'safe' for him to drive home?

Assume:

• Cp of alcohol decreases at 15 mg/100 mL/h
• Vd of alcohol is 50 L
• 100 mL of wine contains 12.5 g alcohol
• driving limit is 80 mg/100 mL.

5 Dosing in renal failure

What maintenance dose of digoxin would be required in a 70-year-old, 70 kg man with a serum creatinine of 0.13 mmol/L, to maintain a serum digoxin concentration of 1 µg/L?

Assume:

• Digoxin cleared entirely renally
• Normal CrCl = 1.5 mL/sec
• The dose in normal renal function is 0.25 mg/day.

6 Dosing in the elderly

What practical dose of quinapril is needed for an 80-year-old, 60 kg woman with serum creatinine of 0.10 mmol/L?

Assume:

- fu quinaprilat (active metabolite) = 0.8
- Usual dose in normal renal function is 20 mg/day
- Tablet size is 5 mg, 10 mg, 20 mg.

7 Dosing in children

If the maintenance dose of a drug for 70 kg adult is 100 mg per day, what is the appropriate dose for a 15 kg child?

8 Drugs and lactation

A 67 kg mother on 100 mg of drug X is breast feeding her 6.7 kg baby. The maternal Cp_{ss} is 1 mg/L.
(i) Calculate the dose of drug the infant will receive.
(ii) Is this compatible with breast feeding?

Assume:

- M/P ratio for drug X = 1
- Milk consumption is 150 mL/kg/day.

9 Drugs/food interaction

Simvastatin is 100% absorbed but only 5% reaches the systemic circulation because of extensive first-pass metabolism. Grapefruit juice totally inhibits this first-pass metabolism, through CYP3A4.

What AUC increase would you expect if grapefruit juice and simvastatin were administered together?

Test Answers

1 Pharmacokinetics

(i)

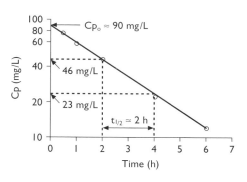

(ii) Estimate Cp_o by back extrapolation

~ 90 mg/L

$$Vd = \frac{Dose}{Cp_o}$$

$$= \frac{1000 \ (mg)}{90 \ (mg/L)}$$

$$= 11.1 \ L$$

(iii) $t_{1/2} = 2$ h (see graph)

(iv) AUC = Sum of trapezoids

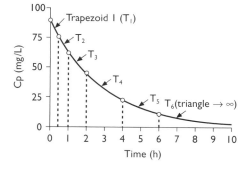

$$T1 = \left(\frac{Cp_o + Cp_{0.5}}{2} \right) \times 0.5 = 42$$

$$T2 = \left(\frac{Cp_{0.5} + Cp_1}{2} \right) \times 0.5 = 35$$

$$T3 = \left(\frac{Cp_1 + Cp_2}{2} \right) \times 1 = 54$$

$$T4 = \left(\frac{Cp_2 + Cp_4}{2} \right) \times 2 = 68$$

$$T5 = \left(\frac{Cp_4 + Cp_6}{2} \right) \times 2 = 34$$

$$T6 = \left(\frac{Cp_6 + 0}{2} \right) \times 6 = 36$$

T6 is a guess to 'infinity', approximated at 12 h

AUC = 42 + 35 + 54 + 68 + 34 + 36 = 269

(v) $Cl = \frac{Dose}{AUC}$

$$= \frac{1000 \ mg}{268 \ (mg/L) \cdot h}$$

$$= 3.72 \ L/h$$

or

$$Cl = \frac{0.693 \times Vd}{t_{1/2}}$$

$$= \frac{0.693 \times 11.1}{2}$$

$$= 3.85 \ L/h$$

2 Loading dose (LD) and maintenance dose (MD)

(i) $LD = Vd \times Cp$
$$= (0.5 \times 50) \quad \times \quad 15$$
$$\quad\quad (L) \quad\quad\quad (mg/L)$$
$$= 375 \text{ mg}$$

(ii) $MD = Cl \times Cp$
$$= (0.04 \times 50) \quad \times \quad 15$$
$$\quad\quad (L/h) \quad\quad\quad (mg/L)$$
$$= 30 \text{ mg/h}$$
$$= 720 \text{ mg/day}$$

3 Dosing in altered metabolism

Intuitive approach

Clearance is doubled $\therefore$ the dose required to achieve Cp of 10 mg/L is double in a smoker.

i.e. 1000 mg/day.
$\therefore$ to achieve 15 mg/L will require 1500 mg/day.

Formal approach

$$MD = Cl \times Cp$$

or $\quad Cl \quad = \dfrac{MD}{Cp}$

$$= \frac{500 \text{ mg/day}}{10 \text{ mg/L}}$$

$$= 50 \text{ L/day}$$

$\therefore$ smokers Cl $\quad = 100$ L/day

$\therefore$ MD (smoker) $= \quad 100 \quad \times \quad 15$
$$\quad\quad\quad (L/day) \quad (mg/L)$$
$$= 1500 \text{ mg/day}$$

4 Saturable kinetics

Calculate maximum Cp possible:

$$Cp = \frac{Dose}{Vd}$$

(from $\quad Ld = Vd \times Cp$)

$$= \frac{12.5 \text{ (L)} \times 8 \text{ (g)}}{50 \text{ (L)}}$$

$$= \frac{100}{50} \text{ g/L}$$

$$= 2 \text{ g/L}$$

$$= 200 \text{ mg/100 mL}$$

To reach 80 mg/100 mL he needs to drop 120 mg/100 mL. At 15 mg/100 mL/h this will take:
$$\frac{120 \text{ mg/100 mL}}{15 \text{ mg/100 mL/h}} = 8h$$

5 Dosing in renal failure

Calculate CrCl, using Cockcroft–Gault equation:

$$CrCl \text{ (mL/s)} = \frac{(140-\text{age}) \times \text{wt (kg)}}{50\,000 \times \text{serum Cr (mmol/L)}}$$

$$= \frac{70 \times 70}{50\,000 \times 0.13}$$

$$= 0.75 \text{ mL}$$

i.e. half normal
$\therefore$ dose is half normal
i.e. 0.125 mg/day

6 Dosing in the elderly

Calculate CrCl using Cockcroft–Gault equation:

$$CrCl(mL/sec) = \left[\frac{(140-80)\times 60}{50\,000 \times 0.10}\right] \times 0.85$$

$$= 0.6 \text{ mL/s}$$

$$\text{Patient dose} = (1-fu) + fu\left(\frac{\text{Patient's CrCl}}{1.5}\right)$$

$$= 0.2 + 0.8\left(\frac{0.6}{1.5}\right)$$

$$= 0.52 \text{ of normal dose}$$

$$\therefore 1 \times 10 \text{ mg tablet per day}$$

7 Dosing in children

Using surface area, SA = 0.62 m²:

$$\text{Maintenance dose} = \frac{SA\ (m^2)}{1.73\ m^2} \times \text{adult dose}$$

$$= \frac{0.62}{1.73} \times 100$$

$$= 36 \text{ mg per day}$$

From weight:

Maintenance dose

$$= \left(\frac{\text{wt (kg)}}{70}\right)^{0.7} \times \text{adult dose}$$

$$= \left(\frac{15}{70}\right)^{0.7} \times 100 \text{ (mg)}$$

$$= 34 \text{ mg per day}$$

8 Drugs and lactation

(i) $\text{Dose}_{\text{infant}} = Cp_{ss}\text{ (mat)} \times M/P \times V_{\text{milk}}$
$$= 1 \times 1 \times (0.15 \times 6.7)$$
$$\quad\ (mg/L)\qquad\quad (L)$$
$$= 1 \text{ mg per day}$$

(ii) This is 1/100 of the maternal dose, but the infant weighs 1/10 of mother's weight. Therefore the infant dose (corrected for weight) is 1/10 the maternal dose. This is right on the notional 10% cut-off level for safety of drugs during breast feeding.

9 Drugs/food interaction

Since the oral availability is only 5%, 95% is metabolized on 'first-pass'. Complete inhibition of this metabolism will increase the oral availability to 100%.

Therefore the AUC will increase 20-fold.

Index